THE OFFICIAL PATIENT'S SOURCEBOOK

on

SARCOIDOSIS

JAMES N. PARKER, M.D.
AND PHILIP M. PARKER, PH.D., EDITORS

ICON Health Publications
ICON Group International, Inc.
4370 La Jolla Village Drive, 4th Floor
San Diego, CA 92122 USA

Last digit indicates print number: 10 9 8 7 6 4 5 3 2 1

Publisher, Health Care: Tiffany LaRochelle
Editor(s): James Parker, M.D., Philip Parker, Ph.D.

Publisher's note: The ideas, procedures, and suggestions contained in this book are not intended as a substitute for consultation with your physician. All matters regarding your health require medical supervision. As new medical or scientific information becomes available from academic and clinical research, recommended treatments and drug therapies may undergo changes. The authors, editors, and publisher have attempted to make the information in this book up to date and accurate in accord with accepted standards at the time of publication. The authors, editors, and publisher are not responsible for errors or omissions or for consequences from application of the book, and make no warranty, expressed or implied, in regard to the contents of this book. Any practice described in this book should be applied by the reader in accordance with professional standards of care used in regard to the unique circumstances that may apply in each situation, in close consultation with a qualified physician. The reader is advised to always check product information (package inserts) for changes and new information regarding dose and contraindications before taking any drug or pharmacological product. Caution is especially urged when using new or infrequently ordered drugs, herbal remedies, vitamins and supplements, alternative therapies, complementary therapies and medicines, and integrative medical treatments.

Cataloging-in-Publication Data

Parker, James N., 1961-
Parker, Philip M., 1960-

   The Official Patient's Sourcebook on Sarcoidosis: A Revised and Updated Directory for the Internet Age/James N. Parker and Philip M. Parker, editors
              p.   cm.
       Includes bibliographical references, glossary and index.
       ISBN: 0-597-83156-4
       1. Sarcoidosis-Popular works.   I. Title.

Disclaimer

This publication is not intended to be used for the diagnosis or treatment of a health problem or as a substitute for consultation with licensed medical professionals. It is sold with the understanding that the publisher, editors, and authors are not engaging in the rendering of medical, psychological, financial, legal, or other professional services.

References to any entity, product, service, or source of information that may be contained in this publication should not be considered an endorsement, either direct or implied, by the publisher, editors or authors. ICON Group International, Inc., the editors, or the authors are not responsible for the content of any Web pages nor publications referenced in this publication.

Copyright Notice

If a physician wishes to copy limited passages from this sourcebook for patient use, this right is automatically granted without written permission from ICON Group International, Inc. (ICON Group). However, all of ICON Group publications are copyrighted. With exception to the above, copying our publications in whole or in part, for whatever reason, is a violation of copyright laws and can lead to penalties and fines. Should you want to copy tables, graphs or other materials, please contact us to request permission (e-mail: iconedit@san.rr.com). ICON Group often grants permission for very limited reproduction of our publications for internal use, press releases, and academic research. Such reproduction requires confirmed permission from ICON Group International Inc. **The disclaimer above must accompany all reproductions, in whole or in part, of this sourcebook.**

Dedication

To the healthcare professionals dedicating their time and efforts to the study of sarcoidosis.

Acknowledgements

The collective knowledge generated from academic and applied research summarized in various references has been critical in the creation of this sourcebook which is best viewed as a comprehensive compilation and collection of information prepared by various official agencies which directly or indirectly are dedicated to sarcoidosis. All of the *Official Patient's Sourcebooks* draw from various agencies and institutions associated with the United States Department of Health and Human Services, and in particular, the Office of the Secretary of Health and Human Services (OS), the Administration for Children and Families (ACF), the Administration on Aging (AOA), the Agency for Healthcare Research and Quality (AHRQ), the Agency for Toxic Substances and Disease Registry (ATSDR), the Centers for Disease Control and Prevention (CDC), the Food and Drug Administration (FDA), the Healthcare Financing Administration (HCFA), the Health Resources and Services Administration (HRSA), the Indian Health Service (IHS), the institutions of the National Institutes of Health (NIH), the Program Support Center (PSC), and the Substance Abuse and Mental Health Services Administration (SAMHSA). In addition to these sources, information gathered from the National Library of Medicine, the United States Patent Office, the European Union, and their related organizations has been invaluable in the creation of this sourcebook. Some of the work represented was financially supported by the Research and Development Committee at INSEAD. This support is gratefully acknowledged. Finally, special thanks are owed to Tiffany LaRochelle for her excellent editorial support.

About the Editors

James N. Parker, M.D.

Dr. James N. Parker received his Bachelor of Science degree in Psychobiology from the University of California, Riverside and his M.D. from the University of California, San Diego. In addition to authoring numerous research publications, he has lectured at various academic institutions. Dr. Parker is the medical editor for the *Official Patient's Sourcebook* series published by ICON Health Publications.

Philip M. Parker, Ph.D.

Philip M. Parker is the Eli Lilly Chair Professor of Innovation, Business and Society at INSEAD (Fontainebleau, France and Singapore). Dr. Parker has also been Professor at the University of California, San Diego and has taught courses at Harvard University, the Hong Kong University of Science and Technology, the Massachusetts Institute of Technology, Stanford University, and UCLA. Dr. Parker is the associate editor for the *Official Patient's Sourcebook* series published by ICON Health Publications.

About ICON Health Publications

In addition to sarcoidosis, *Official Patient's Sourcebooks* are available for the following related topics:

- The Official Patient's Sourcebook on Asthma
- The Official Patient's Sourcebook on Bronchopulmonary Dysplasia
- The Official Patient's Sourcebook on Chronic Obstructive Pulmonary Disease
- The Official Patient's Sourcebook on Cystic Fibrosis
- The Official Patient's Sourcebook on Idiopathic Pulmonary Fibrosis
- The Official Patient's Sourcebook on Primary Pulmonary Hypertension
- The Official Patient's Sourcebook on Pulmonary Lymphangioleiomyomatosis
- The Official Patient's Sourcebook on Respiratory Failure

To discover more about ICON Health Publications, simply check with your preferred online booksellers, including Barnes & Noble.com and Amazon.com which currently carry all of our titles. Or, feel free to contact us directly for bulk purchases or institutional discounts:

ICON Group International, Inc.
4370 La Jolla Village Drive, Fourth Floor
San Diego, CA 92122 USA
Fax: 858-546-4341
Web site: **www.icongrouponline.com/health**

Table of Contents

INTRODUCTION..1
    Overview 1
    Organization 3
    Scope...3
    Moving Forward 4

PART I: THE ESSENTIALS...................................7

CHAPTER 1. THE ESSENTIALS ON SARCOIDOSIS: GUIDELINES............9
    Overview 9
    What Is Sarcoidosis?..11
    Usual Symptoms..11
    Who Gets Sarcoidosis?..12
    Course of the Disease 14
    Diagnosis...15
    Signs and Symptoms..15
    Some Sarcoidosis Sites 16
    Laboratory Tests 17
    Management 19
    Research Status in Sarcoidosis 21
    Living with Sarcoidosis..23
    For More Information 24
    More Guideline Sources...25
    Vocabulary Builder..32

CHAPTER 2. SEEKING GUIDANCE...................................39
    Overview 39
    Associations and Sarcoidosis...................................39
    Finding More Associations 49
    Finding Doctors 51
    Selecting Your Doctor 53
    Working with Your Doctor 53
    Broader Health-Related Resources...........................55
    Vocabulary Builder..55

CHAPTER 3. CLINICAL TRIALS AND SARCOIDOSIS...........................57
    Overview 57
    Recent Trials on Sarcoidosis....................................60
    Benefits and Risks..64

Keeping Current on Clinical Trials 67
General References 68
Vocabulary Builder 68

PART II: ADDITIONAL RESOURCES AND ADVANCED MATERIAL 71

CHAPTER 4. STUDIES ON SARCOIDOSIS 73
Overview 73
The Combined Health Information Database 73
Federally-Funded Research on Sarcoidosis 78
E-Journals: PubMed Central 88
The National Library of Medicine: PubMed 89
Vocabulary Builder 89
CHAPTER 5. PATENTS ON SARCOIDOSIS 93
Overview 93
Patents on Sarcoidosis 94
Patent Applications on Sarcoidosis 98
Keeping Current 98
Vocabulary Builder 99
CHAPTER 6. BOOKS ON SARCOIDOSIS 101
Overview 101
Book Summaries: Federal Agencies 101
The National Library of Medicine Book Index 104
Chapters on Sarcoidosis 107
Directories 112
General Home References 113
Vocabulary Builder 114
CHAPTER 7. MULTIMEDIA ON SARCOIDOSIS 123
Overview 123
Video Recordings 123
Bibliography: Multimedia on Sarcoidosis 124
Vocabulary Builder 126
CHAPTER 8. PERIODICALS AND NEWS ON SARCOIDOSIS 127
Overview 127
News Services & Press Releases 127
Newsletters on Sarcoidosis 130
Newsletter Articles 132
Academic Periodicals covering Sarcoidosis 137

Vocabulary Builder...139
CHAPTER 9. PHYSICIAN GUIDELINES AND DATABASES.................141
   Overview 141
   NIH Guidelines 141
   NIH Databases 144
   Other Commercial Databases 148
   The Genome Project and Sarcoidosis 149
   Specialized References...153
CHAPTER 10. DISSERTATIONS ON SARCOIDOSIS.........................155
   Overview 155
   Dissertations on Sarcoidosis..155
   Keeping Current..156

PART III. APPENDICES **157**

APPENDIX A. RESEARCHING YOUR MEDICATIONS.......................159
   Overview 159
   Your Medications: The Basics 160
   Learning More about Your Medications.............................162
   Commercial Databases..164
   Contraindications and Interactions (Hidden Dangers).......166
   A Final Warning...167
   General References...168
   Vocabulary Builder...168
APPENDIX B. RESEARCHING ALTERNATIVE MEDICINE.................169
   Overview 169
   What Is CAM?..169
   What Are the Domains of Alternative Medicine?...............170
   Can Alternatives Affect My Treatment?...........................173
   Finding CAM References on Sarcoidosis 174
   Additional Web Resources 181
   General References...184
APPENDIX C. RESEARCHING NUTRITION 187
   Overview 187
   Food and Nutrition: General Principles.............................187
   Finding Studies on Sarcoidosis...192
   Federal Resources on Nutrition 196
   Additional Web Resources 196
   Vocabulary Builder...198

APPENDIX D. FINDING MEDICAL LIBRARIES 201
  Overview 201
  Preparation 201
  Finding a Local Medical Library 202
  Medical Libraries Open to the Public 202
APPENDIX E. YOUR RIGHTS AND INSURANCE 209
  Overview 209
  Your Rights as a Patient 209
  Patient Responsibilities 213
  Choosing an Insurance Plan 214
  Medicare and Medicaid 217
  NORD's Medication Assistance Programs 220
  Additional Resources 220
  Vocabulary Builder 221
APPENDIX F. MORE ON THE LUNGS 223
  Overview 223
  Introduction 224
  The Lungs: A Historical View 224
  Human Respiratory System 226
  How Do Normal Lungs Work? 226
  Lung Structure and Function: The Big Picture 227
  The Conducting Airways 228
  Gas Exchange 228
  Cellular and Molecular Aspects 229
APPENDIX G. MORE ON LUNG DISEASES 233
  Overview 233
  How Do Normal Lungs Work? 233
  Lung Diseases: How They Begin 234
  Diseases of the Airways 234
  Diseases of the Interstitium 235
  Disorders of Gas Exchange and Blood Circulation 236
  Disorders of the Pleura 238
  Infections 238
  Early Symptoms of Breathing Problems 239
  Diagnosing Lung Diseases 240
  Spirometry 241
  Treatment 242
  Medications 245

New Developments in Treatment..*247*
The Future *248*

ONLINE GLOSSARIES..**251**
Online Dictionary Directories....................................*260*

SARCOIDOSIS GLOSSARY **261**
General Dictionaries and Glossaries...........................*282*

INDEX **284**

INTRODUCTION

Overview

Dr. C. Everett Koop, former U.S. Surgeon General, once said, "The best prescription is knowledge."[1] The Agency for Healthcare Research and Quality (AHRQ) of the National Institutes of Health (NIH) echoes this view and recommends that every patient incorporate education into the treatment process. According to the AHRQ:

> Finding out more about your condition is a good place to start. By contacting groups that support your condition, visiting your local library, and searching on the Internet, you can find good information to help guide your treatment decisions. Some information may be hard to find — especially if you don't know where to look.[2]

As the AHRQ mentions, finding the right information is not an obvious task. Though many physicians and public officials had thought that the emergence of the Internet would do much to assist patients in obtaining reliable information, in March 2001 the National Institutes of Health issued the following warning:

> The number of Web sites offering health-related resources grows every day. Many sites provide valuable information, while others may have information that is unreliable or misleading.[3]

---

[1] Quotation from **http://www.drkoop.com**.

[2] The Agency for Healthcare Research and Quality (AHRQ):
http://www.ahcpr.gov/consumer/diaginfo.htm.

[3] From the NIH, National Cancer Institute (NCI):
http://cancertrials.nci.nih.gov/beyond/evaluating.html.

Since the late 1990s, physicians have seen a general increase in patient Internet usage rates. Patients frequently enter their doctor's offices with printed Web pages of home remedies in the guise of latest medical research. This scenario is so common that doctors often spend more time dispelling misleading information than guiding patients through sound therapies. *The Official Patient's Sourcebook on Sarcoidosis* has been created for patients who have decided to make education and research an integral part of the treatment process. The pages that follow will tell you where and how to look for information covering virtually all topics related to sarcoidosis, from the essentials to the most advanced areas of research.

The title of this book includes the word "official." This reflects the fact that the sourcebook draws from public, academic, government, and peer-reviewed research. Selected readings from various agencies are reproduced to give you some of the latest official information available to date on sarcoidosis.

Given patients' increasing sophistication in using the Internet, abundant references to reliable Internet-based resources are provided throughout this sourcebook. Where possible, guidance is provided on how to obtain free-of-charge, primary research results as well as more detailed information via the Internet. E-book and electronic versions of this sourcebook are fully interactive with each of the Internet sites mentioned (clicking on a hyperlink automatically opens your browser to the site indicated). Hard copy users of this sourcebook can type cited Web addresses directly into their browsers to obtain access to the corresponding sites. Since we are working with ICON Health Publications, hard copy *Sourcebooks* are frequently updated and printed on demand to ensure that the information provided is current.

In addition to extensive references accessible via the Internet, every chapter presents a "Vocabulary Builder." Many health guides offer glossaries of technical or uncommon terms in an appendix. In editing this sourcebook, we have decided to place a smaller glossary within each chapter that covers terms used in that chapter. Given the technical nature of some chapters, you may need to revisit many sections. Building one's vocabulary of medical terms in such a gradual manner has been shown to improve the learning process.

We must emphasize that no sourcebook on sarcoidosis should affirm that a specific diagnostic procedure or treatment discussed in a research study, patent, or doctoral dissertation is "correct" or your best option. This sourcebook is no exception. Each patient is unique. Deciding on appropriate options is always up to the patient in consultation with their physician and healthcare providers.

Organization

This sourcebook is organized into three parts. Part I explores basic techniques to researching sarcoidosis (e.g. finding guidelines on diagnosis, treatments, and prognosis), followed by a number of topics, including information on how to get in touch with organizations, associations, or other patient networks dedicated to sarcoidosis. It also gives you sources of information that can help you find a doctor in your local area specializing in treating sarcoidosis. Collectively, the material presented in Part I is a complete primer on basic research topics for patients with sarcoidosis.

Part II moves on to advanced research dedicated to sarcoidosis. Part II is intended for those willing to invest many hours of hard work and study. It is here that we direct you to the latest scientific and applied research on sarcoidosis. When possible, contact names, links via the Internet, and summaries are provided. It is in Part II where the vocabulary process becomes important as authors publishing advanced research frequently use highly specialized language. In general, every attempt is made to recommend "free-to-use" options.

Part III provides appendices of useful background reading for all patients with sarcoidosis or related disorders. The appendices are dedicated to more pragmatic issues faced by many patients with sarcoidosis. Accessing materials via medical libraries may be the only option for some readers, so a guide is provided for finding local medical libraries which are open to the public. Part III, therefore, focuses on advice that goes beyond the biological and scientific issues facing patients with sarcoidosis.

Scope

While this sourcebook covers sarcoidosis, your doctor, research publications, and specialists may refer to your condition using a variety of terms. Therefore, you should understand that sarcoidosis is often considered a synonym or a condition closely related to the following:

• Besnier-boeck Disease

• Boeck's Sarcoid

- Erythema Nodosum
- Hilar Adenopathy Plus Uveitis
- Loeffgren's Syndrome
- Sarcoid of Boeck
- Schaumann's Disease

In addition to synonyms and related conditions, physicians may refer to sarcoidosis using certain coding systems. The International Classification of Diseases, 9th Revision, Clinical Modification (ICD-9-CM) is the most commonly used system of classification for the world's illnesses. Your physician may use this coding system as an administrative or tracking tool. The following classification is commonly used for sarcoidosis:[4]

- 135 sarcoidosis

For the purposes of this sourcebook, we have attempted to be as inclusive as possible, looking for official information for all of the synonyms relevant to sarcoidosis. You may find it useful to refer to synonyms when accessing databases or interacting with healthcare professionals and medical librarians.

Moving Forward

Since the 1980s, the world has seen a proliferation of healthcare guides covering most illnesses. Some are written by patients or their family members. These generally take a layperson's approach to understanding and coping with an illness or disorder. They can be uplifting, encouraging, and highly supportive. Other guides are authored by physicians or other healthcare providers who have a more clinical outlook. Each of these two styles of guide has its purpose and can be quite useful.

As editors, we have chosen a third route. We have chosen to expose you to as many sources of official and peer-reviewed information as practical, for the purpose of educating you about basic and advanced knowledge as recognized by medical science today. You can think of this sourcebook as your personal Internet age reference librarian.

---

[4] This list is based on the official version of the World Health Organization's 9th Revision, International Classification of Diseases (ICD-9). According to the National Technical Information Service, "ICD-9CM extensions, interpretations, modifications, addenda, or errata other than those approved by the U.S. Public Health Service and the Health Care Financing Administration are not to be considered official and should not be utilized. Continuous maintenance of the ICD-9-CM is the responsibility of the federal government."

Why "Internet age"? All too often, patients diagnosed with sarcoidosis will log on to the Internet, type words into a search engine, and receive several Web site listings which are mostly irrelevant or redundant. These patients are left to wonder where the relevant information is, and how to obtain it. Since only the smallest fraction of information dealing with sarcoidosis is even indexed in search engines, a non-systematic approach often leads to frustration and disappointment. With this sourcebook, we hope to direct you to the information you need that you would not likely find using popular Web directories. Beyond Web listings, in many cases we will reproduce brief summaries or abstracts of available reference materials. These abstracts often contain distilled information on topics of discussion.

While we focus on the more scientific aspects of sarcoidosis, there is, of course, the emotional side to consider. Later in the sourcebook, we provide a chapter dedicated to helping you find peer groups and associations that can provide additional support beyond research produced by medical science. We hope that the choices we have made give you the most options available in moving forward. In this way, we wish you the best in your efforts to incorporate this educational approach into your treatment plan.

The Editors

PART I: THE ESSENTIALS

ABOUT PART I

Part I has been edited to give you access to what we feel are "the essentials" on sarcoidosis. The essentials of a disease typically include the definition or description of the disease, a discussion of who it affects, the signs or symptoms associated with the disease, tests or diagnostic procedures that might be specific to the disease, and treatments for the disease. Your doctor or healthcare provider may have already explained the essentials of sarcoidosis to you or even given you a pamphlet or brochure describing sarcoidosis. Now you are searching for more in-depth information. As editors, we have decided, nevertheless, to include a discussion on where to find essential information that can complement what your doctor has already told you. In this section we recommend a process, not a particular Web site or reference book. The process ensures that, as you search the Web, you gain background information in such a way as to maximize your understanding.

CHAPTER 1.   THE ESSENTIALS ON SARCOIDOSIS: GUIDELINES

Overview

Official agencies, as well as federally-funded institutions supported by national grants, frequently publish a variety of guidelines on sarcoidosis. These are typically called "Fact Sheets" or "Guidelines." They can take the form of a brochure, information kit, pamphlet, or flyer. Often they are only a few pages in length. The great advantage of guidelines over other sources is that they are often written with the patient in mind. Since new guidelines on sarcoidosis can appear at any moment and be published by a number of sources, the best approach to finding guidelines is to systematically scan the Internet-based services that post them.

The National Institutes of Health (NIH)[5]

The National Institutes of Health (NIH) is the first place to search for relatively current patient guidelines and fact sheets on sarcoidosis. Originally founded in 1887, the NIH is one of the world's foremost medical research centers and the federal focal point for medical research in the United States. At any given time, the NIH supports some 35,000 research grants at universities, medical schools, and other research and training institutions, both nationally and internationally. The rosters of those who have conducted research or who have received NIH support over the years include the world's most illustrious scientists and physicians. Among them are 97 scientists who have won the Nobel Prize for achievement in medicine.

---

[5] Adapted from the NIH: **http://www.nih.gov/about/NIHoverview.html**.

There is no guarantee that any one Institute will have a guideline on a specific disease, though the National Institutes of Health collectively publish over 600 guidelines for both common and rare diseases. The best way to access NIH guidelines is via the Internet. Although the NIH is organized into many different Institutes and Offices, the following is a list of key Web sites where you are most likely to find NIH clinical guidelines and publications dealing with sarcoidosis and associated conditions:

- Office of the Director (OD); guidelines consolidated across agencies available at **http://www.nih.gov/health/consumer/conkey.htm**

- National Library of Medicine (NLM); extensive encyclopedia (A.D.A.M., Inc.) with guidelines available at **http://www.nlm.nih.gov/medlineplus/healthtopics.html**

- National Heart, Lung, and Blood Institute (NHLBI); guidelines at **http://www.nhlbi.nih.gov/guidelines/index.htm**

Among these, the National Heart, Lung, and Blood Institute (NHLBI) is particularly noteworthy. The NHLBI provides leadership for a national program in diseases of the heart, blood vessels, lung, and blood; blood resources; and sleep disorders.[6] Since October 1997, the NHLBI has also had administrative responsibility for the NIH Woman's Health Initiative. The Institute plans, conducts, fosters, and supports an integrated and coordinated program of basic research, clinical investigations and trials, observational studies, and demonstration and education projects. Research is related to the causes, prevention, diagnosis, and treatment of heart, blood vessel, lung, and blood diseases; and sleep disorders. The NHLBI plans and directs research in development and evaluation of interventions and devices related to prevention, treatment, and rehabilitation of patients suffering from such diseases and disorders. It also supports research on clinical use of blood and all aspects of the management of blood resources. Research is conducted in the Institute's own laboratories and by scientific institutions and individuals supported by research grants and contracts. For health professionals and the public, the NHLBI conducts educational activities, including development and dissemination of materials in the above areas, with an emphasis on prevention.

Within the NHLBI, the Division of Lung Diseases (DLD) maintains surveillance over developments in pulmonary research and assesses the Nation's need for research on the causes, prevention, diagnosis, and

---

[6] This paragraph has been adapted from the NHLBI: **http://www.nhlbi.nih.gov/about/org/mission.htm.** "Adapted" signifies that a passage is reproduced exactly or slightly edited for this book.

treatment of pulmonary diseases.[7] Also within the purview of the Division are: technology development, application of research findings, and research training and career development in pulmonary diseases. The DLD plans and directs the research and training programs which encompass basic research, applied research and development, clinical investigations, clinical trials, and demonstration and education research. Two programs comprise the Division of Lung Diseases, Airway Biology and Disease Program, and the Lung Biology and Disease Program. The following patient guideline was recently published by the NHLBI and the DLD on sarcoidosis.

What Is Sarcoidosis?[8]

Sarcoidosis is a disease due to inflammation. It can appear in almost any body organ, but most often starts in the lungs or lymph nodes. No one yet knows what causes sarcoidosis. The disease can appear suddenly and disappear. Or it can develop gradually and go on to produce symptoms that come and go, sometimes for a lifetime.

As sarcoidosis progresses, small lumps, or granulomas, appear in the affected tissues. In the majority of cases, these granulomas clear up, either with or without treatment. In the few cases where the granulomas do not heal and disappear, the tissues tend to remain inflamed and become scarred (fibrotic).

Sarcoidosis was first identified over 100 years ago by two dermatologists working independently, Dr. Jonathan Hutchinson in England and Dr. Caesar Boeck in Norway. Sarcoidosis was originally called Hutchinson's disease or Boeck's disease. Dr. Boeck went on to fashion today's name for the disease from the Greek words "sark" and "oid," meaning flesh-like. The term describes the skin eruptions that are frequently caused by the illness.

Usual Symptoms

Shortness of breath (dyspnea) and a cough that won't go away can be among the first symptoms of sarcoidosis. But sarcoidosis can also show up suddenly with the appearance of skin rashes. Red bumps (erythema nodosum) on the

---

[7] Adapted from the DLD: **http://www.nhlbi.nih.gov/about/dld/index.htm.** For more information, contact: Division of Lung Diseases; National Heart, Lung and Blood Institute; ATTN: Web Site Inquiries; Two Rockledge Center, Suite 10122, 6701 Rockledge Dr., MSC 7952; Bethesda, Maryland 20892-7952.

[8] Adapted from The National Heart Lung And Blood Institute:
http://www.nhlbi.nih.gov/health/public/lung/other/sarcoidosis/index.htm.

face, arms, or shins, and inflammation of the eyes are also common symptoms. It is not unusual, however, for sarcoidosis symptoms to be more general. Weight loss, fatigue, night sweats, fever, or just an overall feeling of ill health can also be clues to the disease.

Who Gets Sarcoidosis?

Sarcoidosis was once considered a rare disease. We now know that it is a common chronic illness that appears all over the world. Indeed, it is the most common of the fibrotic lung disorders, and occurs often enough in the United States for Congress to have declared a national Sarcoidosis Awareness Day in 1990.

Anyone can get sarcoidosis. It occurs in all races and in both sexes. Nevertheless, the risk is greater if you are a young black adult, especially a black woman, or of Scandinavian, German, Irish, or Puerto Rican origin. No one knows why.

Because sarcoidosis can escape diagnosis or be mistaken for several other diseases, we can only guess at how many people are affected. The best estimate today is that about 5 in 100,000 white people in the United States have sarcoidosis. Among black people, it occurs more frequently, in probably 40 out of 100,000 people.

Overall, there appear to be 20 cases per 100,000 in cities on the east coast and somewhat fewer in rural locations. Some scientists, however, believe that these figures greatly underestimated the percentage of the U.S. population with sarcoidosis.

Sarcoidosis mainly affects people between 20 to 40 years of age. White women are just as likely as white men to get sarcoidosis, but the black female gets sarcoidosis two times as often as the black male.

Sarcoidosis also appears to be more common and more severe incertain geographic areas. It has long been recognized as a common disease in Scandinavian countries, where it is estimated to affect 64 out of 100,000 people. But it was not until the mid-1940's--when a large number of cases were identified during mass chest x-ray screening for the Armed Forces--that its high prevalence was recognized in North America.

What Sarcoidosis Is Not

Much about sarcoidosis remains unknown. Nevertheless, if you have the disease, you can be reassured about several things.

- Sarcoidosis is usually not crippling. It often goes away by itself, with most cases healing in 24 to 36 months. Even when sarcoidosis lasts longer, most patients can go about their lives as usual.

- Sarcoidosis is not a cancer. It is not contagious, and your friends and family will not catch it from you.

- Although it can occur in families, there is no evidence that sarcoidosis is passed from parents to children.

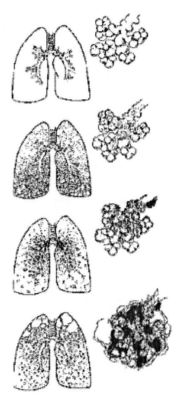

Inflamatory phases in lung sarcoidosis. Magnified views show how illness may affect the normal lung, going from alveolitis, to granuloma formation, to fibrosis.

Some Things We Don't Know about Sarcoidosis

Sarcoidosis is currently thought to be associated with an abnormal immune response. Whether a foreign substance is the trigger; whether that trigger is a chemical, drug, virus, or some other substance; and how exactly the immune disturbance is caused are not known.

Researchers supported by the National Heart, Lung, and Blood Institute are trying to solve some of these mysteries. Among the research questions they are trying to answer are:

- Does sarcoidosis have many causes, or is it produced by a single agent?

- In which body organ does sarcoidosis actually start?

- How does sarcoidosis spread from one part of the body to another?

- Do heredity, environment, and lifestyle play any role in the appearance, severity, or length of the disease?

- Is the abnormal immune response seen in patients a cause or an effect of the disease?

- How can sarcoidosis be prevented?

Course of the Disease

In general, sarcoidosis appears briefly and heals naturally in 60 to 70 percent of the cases, often without the patient knowing or doing anything about it. From 20 to 30 percent of sarcoidosis patients are left with some permanent lung damage. In 10 to 15 percent of the patients, sarcoidosis can become chronic.

When either the granulomas or fibrosis seriously affect the function of a vital organ--the lungs, heart, nervous system, liver, or kidneys, for example--sarcoidosis can be fatal. This occurs 5 to 10 percent of the time.

No one can predict how sarcoidosis will progress in an individual patient. But the symptoms the patient experiences, the doctor's findings, and the patient's race can give some clues.

For example, a sudden onset of general symptoms such as weight loss of feeling poorly are usually taken to mean that the course of sarcoidosis will be relatively short and mild. Dyspnea and possibly skin sarcoidosis often indicate that the sarcoidosis will be more chronic and severe.

White patients are more likely to develop the milder form of the disease while Black patients tend to develop the more chronic and severe form.

Sarcoidosis rarely develops before the age of 10 or after the age of 60. However, the illness--with or without symptoms--has been reported in younger as well as in older people. When symptoms do appear in these age groups, the symptoms are those that are more general in nature, for example, tiredness, sluggishness, coughing and a general feeling of ill health.

Diagnosis

Preliminary diagnosis of sarcoidosis is based on the patient's medical history, routine tests, a physical examination, and a chest x-ray.

The doctor confirms the diagnosis of sarcoidosis by eliminating other diseases with similar features. These include such granulomatous diseases as berylliosis (a disease resulting from exposure to beryllium metal), tuberculosis, farmer's lung disease (hypersensitivity pneumonitis), fungal infections, rheumatoid arthritis, rheumatic fever, and cancer of the lymph nodes (lymphoma).

Signs and Symptoms

In addition to the lungs and lymph nodes, the body organs more likely than others to be affected by sarcoidosis are the liver, skin, heart, nervous system, and kidneys, in that order of frequency. Patients can have symptoms related to the specific organ affected, they can have only general symptoms, or they can be without any symptoms whatsoever. Symptoms also can vary according to how long the illness has been under way, where the granulomas are forming, how much tissue has become affected, and whether the granulomatous process is still active.

Even when there are no symptoms, a doctor can sometimes pick up signs of sarcoidosis during a routine examination, usually a chest x-ray, or when checking out another complaint. The patient's age and race or ethnic group can raise an additional red flag that a sign or symptom of illness could be related to sarcoidosis. Enlargement of the salivary or tear glands and cysts in bone tissue are also among sarcoidosis signals.

Some Sarcoidosis Sites

Lungs

The lungs are usually the first site involved in sarcoidosis. Indeed, about 9 out of 10 sarcoidosis patients have some type of lung problem, with nearly one-third of these patients showing some respiratory symptoms--usually coughing, either dry or with phlegm, and dyspnea. Occasionally, patients have chest pain and a feeling of tightness in the chest.

It is thought that sarcoidosis of the lungs begins with alveolitis (inflammation of the alveoli), the tiny sac like air spaces in the lungs where carbon dioxide and oxygen are exchanged. Alveolitis either clears up spontaneously or leads to granuloma formation. Eventually fibrosis can form, causing the lung to stiffen and making breathing even more difficult.

Eyes

Eye disease occurs in about 20 to 30 percent of patients with sarcoidosis, particularly in children who get the disease. Almost any part of the eye can be affected--the membranes of the eyelids, cornea, outer coat of the eyeball (sclera), retina, and lens. The eye involvement can start with no symptoms at all or with reddening or watery eyes. In a few cases, cataracts, glaucoma, and blindness can result.

Skin

The skin is affected in about 20 percent of sarcoidosis patients. Skin sarcoidosis is usually marked by small, raised patches on the face. Occasionally the patches are purplish in color and larger. Patches can also appear on limbs, face, and buttocks.

Other symptoms include erythema nodosum, mostly on the legs and often accompanied by arthritis in the ankles, elbows, wrists, and hands. Erythema nodosum usually goes away, but other skin problems can persist.

Nervous System

In an occasional case (1 to 5 percent), sarcoidosis can lead to neurological problems. For example, sarcoid granulomas can appear in the brain, spinal cord, and facial and optic nerves. Facial paralysis and other symptoms of nerve damage call for prompt treatment.

Laboratory Tests

No single test can be relied on for a correct diagnosis of sarcoidosis. X-rays and blood tests are usually the first procedures the doctor will order. Pulmonary function tests often provide clues to diagnosis. Other tests may also be used, some more often than others.

Many of the tests that the doctor calls on to help diagnose sarcoidosis can also help the doctor follow the progress of the disease and determine whether the sarcoidosis is getting better or worse.

Chest X-Ray

A picture of the lungs, heart, as well as the surrounding tissues containing lymph nodes, where infection-fighting white blood cells form, can give the first indication of sarcoidosis. For example, a swelling of the lymph glands between the two lungs can show up on an x-ray. An x-ray can also show which areas of the lung are affected.

Pulmonary Function Tests

By performing a variety of tests called pulmonary function tests (PFT), the doctor can find out how well the lungs are doing their job of expanding and exchanging oxygen and carbon dioxide with the blood. The lungs of sarcoidosis patients cannot handle these tasks as well as they should; this is because granulomas and fibrosis of lung tissue decrease lung capacity and disturb the normal flow of gases between the lungs and the blood.

One PFT procedure calls for the patient to breathe into a machine, called a spirometer. It is a mechanical device that records changes in the lung size as air is inhaled and exhaled, as well as the time it takes the patient to do this.

Blood Tests

Blood analyses can evaluate the number and types of blood cells in the body and how well the cells are functioning. They can also measure the levels of various blood proteins known to be involved in immunological activities, and they can show increases in serum calcium levels and abnormal liver function that often accompany sarcoidosis.

Blood tests can measure a blood substance called angiotensin-converting enzyme (ACE). Because the cells that make up granulomas secrete large amounts of ACE, the enzyme levels are often high in patients with sarcoidosis. ACE levels, however, are not always high in sarcoidosis patients, and increased ACE levels can also show up in other illnesses.

Bronchoalveolar Lavage

This test uses an instrument called a bronchoscope--a long, narrow tube with a light at the end--to wash out, or lavage, cells and other materials from inside the lungs. This wash fluid is then examined for the amount of various cells and other substances that reflect inflammation and immune activity in the lungs. A high number of white blood cells in this fluid usually indicates an inflammation in the lungs.

Biopsy

Microscopic examination of specimens of lung tissue obtained with a bronchoscope, or of specimens of other tissues, can tell a doctor where granulomas have formed in the body.

Gallium Scanning

In this procedure, the doctor injects the radioactive chemical element gallium-67 into the patient's vein. The gallium collects at places in the body affected by sarcoidosis and other inflammatory conditions. Two days after the injection, the body is scanned for radioactivity.

Increases in gallium uptake at any site in the body indicate that inflammatory activity has developed at the site and also give an idea of which tissue, and how much tissue, has been affected. However, since any type of inflammation causes gallium uptake, a positive gallium scan does not necessarily mean that the patient has sarcoidosis.

Kveim Test

This test involves injecting a standardized preparation of sarcoid tissue material into the skin. On the one hand, a unique lump formed at the point of injection is considered positive for sarcoidosis. On the other hand, the test result is not always positive even if the patient has sarcoidosis.

The Kveim test is not used often in the United States because no test material has been approved for sale by the U.S. Food and Drug Administration. However, a few hospitals and clinics may have some standardized test preparation prepared privately for their own use.

Slit-Lamp Examination

An instrument called a slit lamp, which permits examination of the inside of the eye, can be used to detect silent damage from sarcoidosis.

Management

Fortunately, many patients with sarcoidosis require no treatment. Symptoms, after all, are usually not disabling and do tend to disappear spontaneously.

When therapy is recommended, the main goal is to keep the lungs and other affected body organs working and to relieve symptoms. The disease is considered inactive once the symptoms fade. After many years of experience with treating the disease, corticosteroids remain the primary treatment for inflammation and granuloma formation. Prednisone is probably the corticosteroid most often prescribed today. There is no treatment at present to reverse the fibrosis that might be present in advanced sarcoidosis.

More than one test is needed to diagnose sarcoidosis. Tests can also show if you are getting better. Occasionally, a blood test will show a high blood level of calcium accompanying sarcoidosis. The reasons for this are not clear. Some scientists believe that this condition is not common. When it does occur, the patient may be advised to avoid calcium-rich foods, vitamin D, or sunlight, or to take prednisone; this corticosteroid quickly reverses the condition.

Because sarcoidosis can disappear even without therapy, doctors sometimes disagree on when to start the treatment, what dose to prescribe, and how long to continue the medicine. The doctor's decision depends on the organ system involved and how far the inflammation has progressed. If the disease appears to be severe-especially in the lungs, eyes, heart, nervous system, spleen, or kidneys-the doctor may prescribe corticosteroids.

Corticosteroid Treatment

Corticosteroid treatment usually results in improvement. Symptoms often start up again, however, when it is stopped. Treatment, therefore, may be necessary for several years, sometimes for as long as the disease remains active or to prevent relapse.

Frequent checkups are important so that the doctor can monitor the illness and, if necessary, adjust the treatment. Corticosteroids, for example, can have side effects-mood swings, swelling, and weight gain because the treatment tends to make the body hold on to water; high blood pressure; high blood sugar; and craving for food. Long-term use can affect the stomach, skin, and bones. This situation can bring on stomach pain, an ulcer, or acne, or cause the loss of calcium from bones. However, if the corticosteroid is taken in carefully prescribed, low doses, the benefits from the treatment are usually far greater than the problems.

Other Drugs

Besides corticosteroids, various other drugs have been tried, but their effectiveness has not been established in controlled studies. These drugs include chloroquine and D-penicillamine.

Several drugs such as chlorambucil, azathioprine, methotrexate, and cyclophosphamide, which might suppress alveolitis by killing the cells that produce granulomas, have also been used. None has been evaluated in controlled clinical trials, and the risk of using these drugs is high, especially in pregnant women.

Cyclosporine, a drug used widely in organ transplants to suppress immune reaction, has been evaluated in one controlled trial. It was found to be unsuccessful.

Research Status in Sarcoidosis

There are many unanswered questions about sarcoidosis. Identifying the agent that causes the illness, along with the inflammatory mechanisms that set the stage for the alveolitis, granuloma formation, and fibrosis that characterize the disease, is the major aim of the National Heart, Lung, and Blood Institute's program on sarcoidosis. Development of reliable methods of diagnosis, treatment, and eventually, the prevention of sarcoidosis is the ultimate goal.

Originally, scientists thought that sarcoidosis was caused by an acquired state of immunological inertness (anergy). This notion was revised a few years ago, when the technique of bronchoalveolar lavage provided access to a vast array of cells and cell-derived mediators operating in the lungs of sarcoidosis patients. Sarcoidosis is now believed to be associated with a complex mix of immunological disturbances involving simultaneous activation, as well as depression, of certain immunological functions.

Immunological studies on sarcoidosis patients show that many of the immune functions associated with thymus-derived white blood cells, called T-lymphocytes or T-cells, are depressed. The depression of this cellular component of systemic immune response is expressed in the inability of the patients to evoke a delayed hypersensitivity skin reaction (a positive skin test), when tested by the appropriate foreign substance, or antigen, underneath the skin.

In addition, the blood of sarcoidosis patients contains a reduced number of T-cells. These T-cells do not seem capable of responding normally when treated with substances known to stimulate the growth of laboratory-cultured T-cells. Neither do they produce their normal complement of immunological mediators, cytokines, through which the cells modify the behavior of other cells.

In contrast to the depression of the cellular immune response, humoral immune response of sarcoidosis patients is elevated. The humoral immune response is reflected by the production of circulating antibodies against a variety of exogenous antigens, including common viruses. This humoral component of systemic immune response is mediated by another class of lymphocytes known as B-lymphocytes, or B-cells, because they originate in the bone marrow.

In another indication of heightened humoral response, sarcoidosis patients seem prone to develop autoantibodies (antibodies against endogenous antigens) similar to rheumatoid factors. With access to the cells and cell products in the lung tissue compartments through the bronchoalveolar technique, it also has become possible for researchers to complement the above investigations at the blood level with analysis of local inflammatory and immune events in the lungs.

In contrast to what is seen at the systemic level, the cellular immune response in the lungs seems to be heightened rather than depressed. The heightened cellular immune response in the diseased tissue is characterized by significant increases in activated T-lymphocytes with certain characteristic cell-surface antigens, as well as in activated alveolar macrophages.

This pronounced, localized cellular response is also accompanied by the appearance in the lung of an array of mediators that are thought to contribute to the disease process; these include interleukin-1, interleukin-2, B-cell growth factor, B-cell differentiation factor, fibroblast growth factor and fibronectin.

Because a number of lung diseases follow respiratory tract infections, ascertaining whether a virus can be implicated in the events leading to sarcoidosis remains an important area of research. Some recent observations seem to provide suggestive leads on this question. In these studies, the genes of cytomegalovirus (CMV), a common disease-causing virus, were introduced into lymphocytes, and the expression of the viral genes was studied. It was found that the viral genes were expressed both during acute infection of the cells and when the virus was not replicating in the cells. However, this expression seemed to take place only when the T-cells were activated by some injurious event.

In addition, the product of a CMV gene was found capable of activating the gene in alveolar macrophage responsible for the production of interleukin-1. Since interleukin-1 levels are found to increase in alveolar macrophage from patients with sarcoidosis, this suggests that certain viral genes can enhance the production of inflammatory components associated with sarcoidosis. Whether these findings implicate viral infections in the disease process in sarcoidosis is unclear. Future research with viral models may provide clues to the molecular mechanisms that trigger alterations in lymphocyte and macrophage regulation leading to sarcoidosis.

In 1995, the National Heart, Lung, and Blood Institute started a multicenter case control study of the etiology of sarcoidosis. The investigation is planned to last six years and will collect information and specimens for use in investigation of environmental, occupational, lifestyle, and genetic risk factors for sarcoidosis. Examination of the natural history of sarcoidosis is planned in patients at early and late stages of the disease. Such information should improve our understanding of the cause(s) of sarcoidosis and provide insight into how to better prevent and treat the disease.

Living with Sarcoidosis

The cause of sarcoidosis still remains unknown, so there is at present no known way to prevent or cure this disease. However, doctors have had a great deal of experience in management of the illness.

If you have sarcoidosis, you can help yourself by following sensible health measures. You should not smoke. You should also avoid exposure to other substances such as dusts and chemicals that can harm your lungs.

Patients with sarcoidosis are best treated by a lung specialist or a doctor who has a special interest in sarcoidosis. Sarcoidosis specialists are usually located at major research centers.

If you have any symptoms of sarcoidosis, see your doctor regularly so that the illness can be watched and, if necessary, treated. If it heals naturally, sarcoidosis is unlikely to recur. Nevertheless, if you have had sarcoidosis, or are suspected of having the illness but have no symptoms now, be sure to have physical checkups every year, including an eye examination.

Although severe sarcoidosis can reduce the chances of becoming pregnant, particularly for older women, many young women with sarcoidosis have given birth to healthy babies while on treatment. Patients planning to have a baby should discuss the matter with their doctor. Medical checkups all through pregnancy and immediately thereafter are especially important for sarcoidosis patients. In some cases, bed rest is necessary during the last 3 months of pregnancy.

In addition to family and close friends, a number of local lung organizations, other nonprofit health organizations, and self-help groups are available to help patients cope with sarcoidosis. By keeping in touch with them, you can share personal feelings and experiences. Members also share specific information on the latest scientific advances, where to find sarcoidosis specialists, and how to improve one's self-image.

For More Information

Additional information on sarcoidosis is available from a number of sources. For the names of U.S. scientists working on sarcoidosis or physicians specializing in the disease, write to:

National Heart, Lung, and Blood Institute
Division of Lung Diseases
2 Rockledge Center
6701 Rockledge Drive
MSC 7952
Suite 10018
Bethesda, MD 20892-7952

If you are interested in participating in clinical studies of sarcoidosis ongoing at the NHLBI, have your physician write to:

National Heart, Lung, and Blood Institute
Pulmonary Branch
9000 Rockville Pike
Building 10, Room 6D06
Bethesda, MD 20892

Information and publications for sarcoidosis patients and their families are available from:

National Institute of Allergy and Infectious Diseases
9000 Rockville Pike
Building 31, Room 7A32
Bethesda, MD 20892

Sarcoidosis Family Aid and Research Foundation
460A Central Avenue
East Orange, NJ 07018

Many local chapters of the American Lung Association host support groups for sarcoidosis patients. The address and telephone number of the chapter nearest to you should be in your local telephone directory. Or you can write or call the association's national headquarters:

American Lung Association
1740 Broadway
New York, NY 10019-4374
(212) 315-8700

Listed below are addresses of organizations that provide additional information and patient support groups on sarcoidosis:

Sarcoidosis Networking
13925 80th Street East
Puyallup, WA 98372
(206) 845-3108

National Sarcoidosis Resources Center
P.O. Box 1593
Piscataway, NJ 08855-1593
(908) 699-0733

Sarcoidosis Research Institute
3475 Central Avenue
Memphis, TN 38111
(901) 327-5454

More Guideline Sources

The guideline above on sarcoidosis is only one example of the kind of material that you can find online and free of charge. The remainder of this chapter will direct you to other sources which either publish or can help you find additional guidelines on topics related to sarcoidosis. Many of the guidelines listed below address topics that may be of particular relevance to your specific situation or of special interest to only some patients with sarcoidosis. Due to space limitations these sources are listed in a concise manner. Do not hesitate to consult the following sources by either using the Internet hyperlink provided, or, in cases where the contact information is provided, contacting the publisher or author directly.

Topic Pages: MEDLINEplus

For patients wishing to go beyond guidelines published by specific Institutes of the NIH, the National Library of Medicine has created a vast and patient-oriented healthcare information portal called MEDLINEplus. Within this Internet-based system are "health topic pages." You can think of a health topic page as a guide to patient guides. To access this system, log on to **http://www.nlm.nih.gov/medlineplus/healthtopics.html**. From there you can either search using the alphabetical index or browse by broad topic areas. Recently, MEDLINEplus listed the following as being relevant to sarcoidosis:

- Guides on sarcoidosis

  Sarcoidosis
  http://www.nlm.nih.gov/medlineplus/ency/article/000076.htm

  Sarcoidosis
  http://www.nlm.nih.gov/medlineplus/sarcoidosis.html

  Sarcoidosis
  http://www.nlm.nih.gov/medlineplus/tutorials/sacroidosisloader.html

- Other guides

  Neurosarcoidosis
  http://www.nlm.nih.gov/medlineplus/ency/article/000720.htm

  Pulmonary tuberculosis
  http://www.nlm.nih.gov/medlineplus/ency/article/000077.htm

  Erythema nodosum
  http://www.nlm.nih.gov/medlineplus/ency/article/000881.htm

  Disseminated tuberculosis
  http://www.nlm.nih.gov/medlineplus/ency/article/000624.htm

  Uveitis
  http://www.nlm.nih.gov/medlineplus/ency/article/001005.htm

  Diffuse interstitial pulmonary fibrosis
  http://www.nlm.nih.gov/medlineplus/ency/article/000128.htm

Within the health topic page dedicated to sarcoidosis, the following was recently recommended to patients:

- General/Overviews

  Living With Sarcoidosis
  Source: American Medical Association
  http://www.ama-assn.org/public/journals/patient/archive/jpg031302.htm

Sarcoidosis

http://www.nlm.nih.gov/medlineplus/tutorials/sacroidosisloader.html

Sarcoidosis

Source: American Academy of Family Physicians

http://familydoctor.org/handouts/320.html

<u>Sarcoidosis</u>

Source: American Lung Association

http://www.lungusa.org/diseases/lungsarcoido.html

Sarcoidosis

Source: Arthritis Foundation

http://www.arthritis.org/conditions/DiseaseCenter/sarcoidosis.asp

Sarcoidosis

Source: Mayo Foundation for Medical Education and Research

http://www.mayoclinic.com/invoke.cfm?id=DS00251

- Specific Conditions/Aspects

  Minority Lung Disease Data: Sarcoidosis

  Source: American Lung Association

  http://www.lungusa.org/pub/minority/sarcoidosis.html

- From the National Institutes of Health

  Sarcoidosis

  Source: National Heart, Lung, and Blood Institute

  http://www.nhlbi.nih.gov/health/public/lung/other/sarcoidosis/index.htm

- Organizations

  American Lung Association

  http://www.lungusa.org/index.html

  Arthritis Foundation

  http://www.arthritis.org/

  National Heart, Lung, and Blood Institute

  http://www.nhlbi.nih.gov/index.htm

If you do not find topics of interest when browsing health topic pages, then you can choose to use the advanced search utility of MEDLINEplus at **http://www.nlm.nih.gov/medlineplus/advancedsearch.html**. This utility is similar to the NIH Search Utility, with the exception that it only includes material linked within the MEDLINEplus system (mostly patient-oriented information). It also has the disadvantage of generating unstructured results. We recommend, therefore, that you use this method only if you have a very targeted search.

The Combined Health Information Database (CHID)

CHID Online is a reference tool that maintains a database directory of thousands of journal articles and patient education guidelines on sarcoidosis and related conditions. One of the advantages of CHID over other sources is that it offers summaries that describe the guidelines available, including contact information and pricing. CHID's general Web site is **http://chid.nih.gov/**. To search this database, go to **http://chid.nih.gov/detail/detail.html**. In particular, you can use the advanced search options to look up pamphlets, reports, brochures, and information kits. The following was recently posted in this archive:

- **Facts About Sarcoidosis**

  Source: Sumner, WA: Sarcoid Networking Association. 2000. 6 p.

  Contact: Available from Sarcoid Networking Association. 6424 151st Avenue East, Sumner, WA 98390-2601. (253) 891-6886. E-mail: sarcoidosis_network@prodigy.net. PRICE: Single copy free.

  Summary: This pamphlet uses a question and answer format to provide people who have sarcoidosis with information on the etiology, symptoms, diagnosis, and treatment of this multisystem, granulomatous disease. Although the cause of sarcoidosis in unknown, possible causes include a viral or bacterial infection, an immune system defect, exposure to a toxic substance, an unknown environmental trigger, and an inherited or genetic factor. The disease affects all races and age groups. Symptoms depend on the organ with granulomas. Diagnosis is based on physical examination and diagnostic test findings. If symptoms do not resolve without treatment, therapeutic options include corticosteroids and immune suppressants. 1 figure.

- **Answers to Your Questions About Sarcoidosis**

  Source: Memphis, TN: Sarcoidosis Research Institute. 8 p.

  Contact: Available from Sarcoidosis Research Institute. 3475 Central Avenue, Memphis, TN 38111. (901) 766-6951 or (901) 452- 1470. Price: Free.

Summary: This brochure answers commonly asked questions about sarcoidosis. Information includes a general description of the disease, diagnosis, symptoms, treatments and information on the Sarcoidosis Research Institute.

The National Guideline Clearinghouse™

The National Guideline Clearinghouse™ offers hundreds of evidence-based clinical practice guidelines published in the United States and other countries. You can search their site located at **http://www.guideline.gov** by using the keyword "sarcoidosis" or synonyms. The following was recently posted:

- **Clinical practice guidelines for the use of chemotherapy and radiotherapy protectants.**

  Source: American Society of Clinical Oncology.; 1999 October; 23 pages

  http://www.guideline.gov/FRAMESETS/guideline_fs.asp?guideline=001376&sSearch_string=sarcoidosis

- **Dry eye syndrome.**

  Source: American Academy of Ophthalmology.; 1998 September; 18 pages

  http://www.guideline.gov/FRAMESETS/guideline_fs.asp?guideline=000739&sSearch_string=sarcoidosis

- **Heart failure.**

  Source: American Medical Directors Association.; 1996; 12 pages

  http://www.guideline.gov/FRAMESETS/guideline_fs.asp?guideline=001035&sSearch_string=sarcoidosis

- **Practice guidelines for diseases caused by Aspergillus.**

  Source: Infectious Diseases Society of America.; 2000 April; 14 pages

  http://www.guideline.gov/FRAMESETS/guideline_fs.asp?guideline=001893&sSearch_string=sarcoidosis

- **Practice guidelines for the management of community-acquired pneumonia in adults.**

  Source: Infectious Diseases Society of America.; 2000 February; 36 pages

  http://www.guideline.gov/FRAMESETS/guideline_fs.asp?guideline=00 1891&sSearch_string=sarcoidosis

- **Procedure guideline for gallium scintigraphy in inflammation.**

  Source: Society of Nuclear Medicine, Inc..; 1999 February; 21 pages

  http://www.guideline.gov/FRAMESETS/guideline_fs.asp?guideline=00 0607&sSearch_string=sarcoidosis

- **Single-breath carbon monoxide diffusing capacity, 1999 update.**

  Source: American Association for Respiratory Care.; 1999 January; 9 pages

  http://www.guideline.gov/FRAMESETS/guideline_fs.asp?guideline=00 0993&sSearch_string=sarcoidosis

- **VHA/DOD clinical practice guideline for the management of major depressive disorder in adults.**

  Source: Department of Veterans Affairs/Veterans Health Administration.; 1997 (updated 2000); Various pagings

  http://www.guideline.gov/FRAMESETS/guideline_fs.asp?guideline=00 1811&sSearch_string=sarcoidosis

Healthfinder™

Healthfinder™ is an additional source sponsored by the U.S. Department of Health and Human Services which offers links to hundreds of other sites that contain healthcare information. This Web site is located at **http://www.healthfinder.gov**. Again, keyword searches can be used to find guidelines. The following was recently found in this database:

- **Sarcoidosis**

  Summary: Information on what is know and not know about sarcoidosis, the most common of the fibrotic lung disorders. The symptoms, course of the disease, diagnosis, and management are discussed.

  Source: National Heart, Lung, and Blood Institute, National Institutes of Health

  http://www.healthfinder.gov/scripts/recordpass.asp?RecordType=0&RecordID=723

The NIH Search Utility

After browsing the references listed at the beginning of this chapter, you may want to explore the NIH Search Utility. This allows you to search for documents on over 100 selected Web sites that comprise the NIH-WEB-SPACE. Each of these servers is "crawled" and indexed on an ongoing basis. Your search will produce a list of various documents, all of which will relate in some way to sarcoidosis. The drawbacks of this approach are that the information is not organized by theme and that the references are often a mix of information for professionals and patients. Nevertheless, a large number of the listed Web sites provide useful background information. We can only recommend this route, therefore, for relatively rare or specific disorders, or when using highly targeted searches. To use the NIH search utility, visit the following Web page: **http://search.nih.gov/index.html**.

NORD (The National Organization of Rare Disorders, Inc.)

NORD provides an invaluable service to the public by publishing, for a nominal fee, short yet comprehensive guidelines on over 1,000 diseases. NORD primarily focuses on rare diseases that might not be covered by the previously listed sources. NORD's Web address is **www.rarediseases.org**. To see if a recent fact sheet has been published on sarcoidosis, simply go to the following hyperlink: **http://www.rarediseases.org/cgi-bin/nord/alphalist**. A complete guide on sarcoidosis can be purchased from NORD for a nominal fee.

Additional Web Sources

A number of Web sites that often link to government sites are available to the public. These can also point you in the direction of essential information. The following is a representative sample:

- AOL: **http://search.aol.com/cat.adp?id=168&layer=&from=subcats**

- drkoop.com®: **http://www.drkoop.com/conditions/ency/index.html**

- Family Village: **http://www.familyvillage.wisc.edu/specific.htm**

- Google: **http://directory.google.com/Top/Health/Conditions_and_Diseases/**

- Med Help International: **http://www.medhelp.org/HealthTopics/A.html**

- Open Directory Project: **http://dmoz.org/Health/Conditions_and_Diseases/**

- Yahoo.com: **http://dir.yahoo.com/Health/Diseases_and_Conditions/**

- WebMD®Health: **http://my.webmd.com/health_topics**

Vocabulary Builder

The material in this chapter may have contained a number of unfamiliar words. The following Vocabulary Builder introduces you to terms used in this chapter that have not been covered in the previous chapter:

Acne: An inflammatory disease of the pilosebaceous unit, the specific type usually being indicated by a modifying term; frequently used alone to designate common acne, or acne vulgaris. [EU]

Alveolitis: Inflammation of the alveoli. [NIH]

Anergy: Absence of immune response to particular substances. [NIH]

Ankle: That part of the lower limb directly above the foot. [NIH]

Antibodies: Specific proteins produced by the body's immune system that bind with foreign proteins (antigens). [NIH]

Antigen: Any substance which is capable, under appropriate conditions, of inducing a specific immune response and of reacting with the products of that response, that is, with specific antibody or specifically sensitized T-lymphocytes, or both. Antigens may be soluble substances, such as toxins and foreign proteins, or particulate, such as bacteria and tissue cells; however, only the portion of the protein or polysaccharide molecule known as the antigenic determinant (q.v.) combines with antibody or a specific receptor on a lymphocyte. Abbreviated Ag. [EU]

Aspergillus: A genus of mitosporic fungi containing about 100 species and eleven different teleomorphs in the family Trichocomaceae. [NIH]

Berylliosis: A lung disease resulting from exposure to beryllium metal. [NIH]

Beryllium: Beryllium. An element with the atomic symbol Be, atomic number 4, and atomic weight 9.01218. Short exposure to this element can lead to a type of poisoning known as berylliosis. [NIH]

Biopsy: The removal and examination, usually microscopic, of tissue from the living body, performed to establish precise diagnosis. [EU]

Blindness: The inability to see or the loss or absence of perception of visual stimuli. This condition may be the result of eye diseases; optic nerve diseases; optic chiasm diseases; or brain diseases affecting the visual pathways or occipital lobe. [NIH]

Bronchoscope: A long, narrow tube with a light at the end that is used by the doctor for direct observation of the airways, as well as for suction of tissue and other materials. [NIH]

Cataract: An opacity, partial or complete, of one or both eyes, on or in the lens or capsule, especially an opacity impairing vision or causing blindness. The many kinds of cataract are classified by their morphology (size, shape, location) or etiology (cause and time of occurrence). [EU]

Cell: Basic subunit of every living organism; the simplest unit that can exist as an independent living system. [NIH]

Chemotherapy: The treatment of disease by means of chemicals that have a specific toxic effect upon the disease - producing microorganisms or that selectively destroy cancerous tissue. [EU]

Chloroquine: The prototypical antimalarial agent with a mechanism that is not well understood. It has also been used to treat rheumatoid arthritis, systemic lupus erythematosus, and in the systemic therapy of amebic liver abscesses. [NIH]

Chronic: Of long duration; frequently recurring. [NIH]

Cornea: The transparent structure forming the anterior part of the fibrous tunic of the eye. It consists of five layers : (1) the anterior corneal epithelium, continuous with that of the conjunctiva, (2) the anterior limiting layer (Bowman's membrane), (3) the substantia propria, or stroma, (4) the posterior limiting layer (Descemet's membrane), and (5) the endothelium of the anterior chamber, called also keratoderma. [EU]

Corticosteroids: Drugs that mimic the action of a group of hormones produced by adrenal glands; they are anti-inflammatory and act as bronchodilators. [NIH]

Cyclophosphamide: Precursor of an alkylating nitrogen mustard antineoplastic and immunosuppressive agent that must be activated in the liver to form the active aldophosphamide. It is used in the treatment of lymphomas, leukemias, etc. Its side effect, alopecia, has been made use of in defleecing sheep. Cyclophosphamide may also cause sterility, birth defects, mutations, and cancer. [NIH]

Cyst: Any closed cavity or sac; normal or abnormal, lined by epithelium, and especially one that contains a liquid or semisolid material. [EU]

Cytokines: Non-antibody proteins secreted by inflammatory leukocytes and some non-leukocytic cells, that act as intercellular mediators. They differ from classical hormones in that they are produced by a number of tissue or cell types rather than by specialized glands. They generally act locally in a paracrine or autocrine rather than endocrine manner. [NIH]

Cytomegalovirus: A genus of the family herpesviridae, subfamily betaherpesvirinae, infecting the salivary glands, liver, spleen, lungs, eyes, and other organs, in which they produce characteristically enlarged cells with intranuclear inclusions. Infection with Cytomegalovirus is also seen as an opportunistic infection in AIDS. [NIH]

Dyspnea: Shortness of breath; difficult or labored breathing. [NIH]

Endogenous: Developing or originating within the organisms or arising from causes within the organism. [EU]

Enzyme: Substance, made by living cells, that causes specific chemical changes. [NIH]

Erythema: A name applied to redness of the skin produced by congestion of the capillaries, which may result from a variety of causes, the etiology or a specific type of lesion often being indicated by a modifying term. [EU]

Exogenous: Developed or originating outside the organism, as exogenous disease. [EU]

Fatal: Causing death, deadly; mortal; lethal. [EU]

Fatigue: The state of weariness following a period of exertion, mental or physical, characterized by a decreased capacity for work and reduced efficiency to respond to stimuli. [NIH]

Fibrosis: Process by which inflamed tissue becomes scarred. [NIH]

Gallium: A rare, metallic element designated by the symbol, Ga, atomic number 31, and atomic weight 69.72. [NIH]

Genitourinary: Pertaining to the genital and urinary organs; urogenital; urinosexual. [EU]

Granulomas: Small lumps in tissues caused by inflammation. [NIH]

Heredity: 1. the genetic transmission of a particular quality or trait from parent to offspring. 2. the genetic constitution of an individual. [EU]

Humoral: Of, relating to, proceeding from, or involving a bodily humour - now often used of endocrine factors as opposed to neural or somatic. [EU]

Hypersensitivity: A state of altered reactivity in which the body reacts with an exaggerated immune response to a foreign substance. Hypersensitivity reactions are classified as immediate or delayed, types I and IV, respectively, in the Gell and Coombs classification (q.v.) of immune responses. [EU]

Inflammation: Response of the body tissues to injury; typical signs are swelling, redness, and pain. [NIH]

Interstitial: Pertaining to or situated between parts or in the interspaces of a tissue. [EU]

Lavage: To wash the interior of a body organ. [NIH]

Lymph: A transparent, slightly yellow liquid found in the lymphatic vessels. Lymph is collected from tissue fluids throughout the body and returned to the blood via the lymphatic system. [NIH]

Lymphoma: Cancer of the lymph nodes. [NIH]

Mediator: An object or substance by which something is mediated, such as (1) a structure of the nervous system that transmits impulses eliciting a specific response; (2) a chemical substance (transmitter substance) that induces activity in an excitable tissue, such as nerve or muscle; or (3) a substance released from cells as the result of the interaction of antigen with antibody or by the action of antigen with a sensitized lymphocyte. [EU]

Membrane: Thin, flexible film of proteins and lipids that encloses the contents of a cell; it controls the substances that go into and come out of the cell. Also, a thin layer of tissue that covers the surface or lines the cavity of an organ. [NIH]

Methotrexate: An antineoplastic antimetabolite with immunosuppressant properties. It is an inhibitor of dihydrofolate reductase and prevents the formation of tetrahydrofolate, necessary for synthesis of thymidylate, an essential component of DNA. [NIH]

Molecular: Of, pertaining to, or composed of molecules : a very small mass of matter. [EU]

Ophthalmology: A surgical specialty concerned with the structure and function of the eye and the medical and surgical treatment of its defects and diseases. [NIH]

Optic: Of or pertaining to the eye. [EU]

Paralysis: Loss or impairment of motor function in a part due to lesion of the neural or muscular mechanism; also by analogy, impairment of sensory function (sensory paralysis). In addition to the types named below, paralysis is further distinguished as traumatic, syphilitic, toxic, etc., according to its cause; or as obturator, ulnar, etc., according to the nerve part, or muscle specially affected. [EU]

Penicillamine: 3-Mercapto-D-valine. The most characteristic degradation product of the penicillin antibiotics. It is used as an antirheumatic and as a chelating agent in Wilson's disease. [NIH]

PFT: Pulmonary function test. [NIH]

Pneumonia: Inflammation of the lungs. [NIH]

Pneumonitis: A disease caused by inhaling a wide variety of substances such as dusts and molds. Also called "farmer's disease". [NIH]

Prednisone: A synthetic anti-inflammatory glucocorticoid derived from cortisone. It is biologically inert and converted to prednisolone in the liver. [NIH]

Proteins: Polymers of amino acids linked by peptide bonds. The specific sequence of amino acids determines the shape and function of the protein. [NIH]

Pulmonary: Relating to the lungs. [NIH]

Radioactivity: The quality of emitting or the emission of corpuscular or electromagnetic radiations consequent to nuclear disintegration, a natural property of all chemical elements of atomic number above 83, and possible of induction in all other known elements. [EU]

Radiology: A specialty concerned with the use of x-ray and other forms of radiant energy in the diagnosis and treatment of disease. [NIH]

Radiotherapy: The treatment of disease by ionizing radiation. [EU]

Respiratory: Pertaining to respiration. [EU]

Retina: The inner layer of tissue at the back of the eye that is sensitive to light. [NIH]

Rheumatoid: Resembling rheumatism. [EU]

Sarcoidosis: An idiopathic systemic inflammatory granulomatous disorder comprised of epithelioid and multinucleated giant cells with little necrosis. It usually invades the lungs with fibrosis and may also involve lymph nodes, skin, liver, spleen, eyes, phalangeal bones, and parotid glands. [NIH]

Sclera: Outer coat of the eyeball. [NIH]

Serum: The clear portion of any body fluid; the clear fluid moistening serous membranes. 2. blood serum; the clear liquid that separates from blood on clotting. 3. immune serum; blood serum from an immunized animal used for passive immunization; an antiserum; antitoxin, or antivenin. [EU]

Stomach: An organ of digestion situated in the left upper quadrant of the abdomen between the termination of the esophagus and the beginning of the duodenum. [NIH]

Sweat: The fluid excreted by the sweat glands. It consists of water containing sodium chloride, phosphate, urea, ammonia, and other waste products. [NIH]

Systemic: Relating to a process that affects the body generally; in this instance, the way in which blood is supplied through the aorta to all body organs except the lungs. [NIH]

Toxic: Pertaining to, due to, or of the nature of a poison or toxin; manifesting the symptoms of severe infection. [EU]

Tuberculosis: Any of the infectious diseases of man and other animals caused by species of mycobacterium. [NIH]

Ulcer: A local defect, or excavation, of the surface of an organ or tissue; which is produced by the sloughing of inflammatory necrotic tissue. [EU]

Uveitis: An inflammation of part or all of the uvea, the middle (vascular) tunic of the eye, and commonly involving the other tunics (the sclera and cornea, and the retina). [EU]

Vein: Vessel-carrying blood from various parts of the body to the heart. [NIH]

Venereal: Pertaining or related to or transmitted by sexual contact. [EU]

Viral: Pertaining to, caused by, or of the nature of virus. [EU]

Viruses: Minute infectious agents whose genomes are composed of DNA or RNA, but not both. They are characterized by a lack of independent metabolism and the inability to replicate outside living host cells. [NIH]

CHAPTER 2. SEEKING GUIDANCE

Overview

Some patients are comforted by the knowledge that a number of organizations dedicate their resources to helping people with sarcoidosis. These associations can become invaluable sources of information and advice. Many associations offer aftercare support, financial assistance, and other important services. Furthermore, healthcare research has shown that support groups often help people to better cope with their conditions.[9] In addition to support groups, your physician can be a valuable source of guidance and support. Therefore, finding a physician that can work with your unique situation is a very important aspect of your care.

In this chapter, we direct you to resources that can help you find patient organizations and medical specialists. We begin by describing how to find associations and peer groups that can help you better understand and cope with sarcoidosis. The chapter ends with a discussion on how to find a doctor that is right for you.

Associations and Sarcoidosis

As mentioned by the Agency for Healthcare Research and Quality, sometimes the emotional side of an illness can be as taxing as the physical side.[10] You may have fears or feel overwhelmed by your situation. Everyone has different ways of dealing with disease or physical injury. Your attitude,

---

[9] Churches, synagogues, and other houses of worship might also have groups that can offer you the social support you need.
[10] This section has been adapted from http://www.ahcpr.gov/consumer/diaginf5.htm.

your expectations, and how well you cope with your condition can all influence your well-being. This is true for both minor conditions and serious illnesses. For example, a study on female breast cancer survivors revealed that women who participated in support groups lived longer and experienced better quality of life when compared with women who did not participate. In the support group, women learned coping skills and had the opportunity to share their feelings with other women in the same situation.

In addition to associations or groups that your doctor might recommend, we suggest that you consider the following list (if there is a fee for an association, you may want to check with your insurance provider to find out if the cost will be covered):

- **American Academy of Allergy Asthma and Immunology**

    Address: American Academy of Allergy Asthma and Immunology 611 East Wells Street, Milwaukee, WI 53202

    Telephone: (414) 272-6071 Toll-free: (800) 822-2762

    Fax: (414) 276-3349

    Email: info@aaaai.org

    Web Site: http://www.aaaai.org

    Background: The American Academy of Allergy, Asthma and Immunology (AAAAI) is an international, not-for-profit professional medical specialty organization representing allergists, clinical immunologists, allied health professionals, and other physicians with a special interest in allergy and immunology. Established in 1943 by the merger of the American Association for the Study of Allergy and the Association for the Study of Asthma and Allied Conditions, the AAAAI is dedicated to advancing the knowledge and practice of allergy, fostering the education of students and the public, encouraging union and cooperation among those working in the field, and promoting and stimulating research and the study of allergic diseases. The AAAAI is currently organized into several major 'interest sections' consisting of Asthma, Rhinitis, and Other Respiratory Diseases; Basic and Clinical Immunology; Dermatologic Diseases; Environmental and Occupational Disorders; Food and Drug Reactions and Anaphylaxis; and Mechanisms of Allergy. The AAAAI also engages in patient advocacy and lobbying activities, provides physician referrals, engages in patient education, and provides a variety of informational materials. The Academy currently has more than 5,400 members in the United States, Canada, and over 40 additional countries.

    Relevant area(s) of interest: Sarcoidosis

- **American Autoimmune Related Diseases Association, Inc**

  Address: American Autoimmune Related Diseases Association, Inc. Michigan National Bank Building, 15475 Gratiot Avenue, Detroit, MI 48205

  Telephone: (313) 371-8600 Toll-free: (800) 598- 4668

  Fax: (313) 371-6002

  Email: aarda@aol.com

  Web Site: http://www.aarda.org/

  Background: The American Autoimmune Related Diseases Association, Inc. (AARDA) is a national not-for-profit voluntary health agency dedicated to bringing a national focus to autoimmunity, a major cause of serious chronic diseases. The Association was founded for the purposes of supporting research to find a cure for autoimmune diseases and providing services to affected individuals. In addition, the Association's goals include increasing the public's awareness that autoimmunity is the cause of more than 80 serious chronic diseases; bringing national focus and collaborative effort among state and national voluntary health groups that represent autoimmune diseases; and serving as a national advocate for individuals and families affected by the physical, emotional, and financial effects of autoimmune disease. The American Autoimmune Related Diseases Association produces educational and support materials including fact sheets, brochures, pamphlets, and a newsletter entitled 'In Focus.'.

  Relevant area(s) of interest: Sarcoidosis

- **American Liver Foundation**

  Address: American Liver Foundation 75 Maiden Lane, Suite 603, New York, NY 10038

  Telephone: (212) 668-1000 Toll-free: (800) 465-4837

  Fax: (973) 256-321

  Email: webmail@liverfoundation.org

  Web Site: http://www.liverfoundation.org

  Background: The American Liver Foundation is a national voluntary not-for-profit organization dedicated to the prevention, treatment, and cure of diseases of the liver through programs of research and education. Established in 1976, the Foundation's activities include support groups, patient advocacy, support of medical research, and patient and professional education. Educational materials include brochures on Hepatitis, Cirrhosis, Biliary Atresia, liver transplantation, gallstones, and

Hereditary Hemochromatosis. Fact sheets are also available on a variety of liver diseases including Alagille Syndrome, Alpha-1-Antitrypsin Deficiency, Cancer of the Liver, Fatty Liver, Gilbert Syndrome, Primary Biliary Cirrhosis, Porphyria, and others. Videotapes produced by the Foundation include 'A Healthy Liver: A Happier Life,' 'Foundations for Decision Making,' 'Hepatitis B: Patient Information,' 'Hepatitis C: A Guide for Primary Care Physicians,' and 'The Visionaries.' The Foundation also offers liver wellness and substance abuse prevention programs to elementary schools and corporations.

Relevant area(s) of interest: Sarcoidosis

- **American Lung Association of Washington**

  Address: 2625 Third Avenue Seattle, WA, 98121

  Telephone: (206) 441-3277 FAX; (206) 441-5100 Voice(800) 732-9339 Voice

  Background: A non-profit organization, the American Lung Association of Washington leads the fight to prevent lung disease and promote lung health through education, community service, research and advocacy. Our four offices around the state focus on reducing tobacco use, especially among young people; preventing indoor and outdoor air pollution; funding research to find the causes of and cures for lung disease; and providing education,information, and services to help people with asthma or other lung disease and their families.

  Relevant area(s) of interest: Adolescents And Young Adults; Air Pollution; All Ages; Asthma; Bronchitis; Consumer Resources; Emphysema; Funding Sources; Indoor Air Quality; Infants; Lung Cancer; Lung Disease; Minority Health; Pneumonia; Respiratory Diseases; Sarcoidosis; Tobacco; Toll-Free Information Services; Tuberculosis

- **Australian Lung Foundation**

  Address: Australian Lung Foundation PO Box 119, Samford, Queensland, 4520, Australia

  Telephone: 07 3832 2245 Toll-free: 1800 654 301

  Fax: 07 3832 145

  Email: alfnat@ozemail.com.au

  Web Site: http://www.lungnet.org.au

  Background: The Australian Lung Foundation (ALF) is a not-for-profit organization that is committed to improving the quality of life of individuals affected by lung disease and promoting lung health in Australia. Established in 1990, the Foundation works to fulfill its mission by raising funds in support of lung disease research, distributing research findings, educating patients and the broader public on the treatment and prevention of lung disease, fostering patient support activities, and influencing public and corporate policy to ensure safe living and working environments. The ALF's activities include providing annual research grants and awards; working with industries to enhance employee safety and corporate productivity; and conducting conferences that are open to all members of the respiratory and wider medical community, government and corporate bodies, special interest groups, and patient support organizations. The Foundation's objectives include establishing the ALF Collaborative Research Institute to facilitate cooperative research and interaction both nationally and internationally and provide a centralized data collection site for respiratory disease; creating multidisciplinary consultative groups to enhance collaboration, generate educational material, and provide a source of expert opinion and comment on lung disease issues; and establishing a national network of patient support groups. The Foundation also provides educational materials including patient information leaflets and maintains a web site on the Internet.

Relevant area(s) of interest: Sarcoidosis

- **British Lung Foundation**

Address: British Lung Foundation 78 Hatton Garden, London, EC1N 8JR, United Kingdom

Telephone: 0171 831 5831

Fax: 0171 831 5832

Email: blf_user@gpiag-asthma.org

Web Site: http://www.lunguk.org/index.htm

Background: The British Lung Foundation is a voluntary, not-for-profit organization in the United Kingdom dedicated to funding medical research into the prevention, treatment, and cure of all forms of lung disease. Since the Foundation was founded in 1985, it has funded over 220 clinical, non-clinical, and epidemiological research grants. The British Lung Foundation is also committed to providing information, support, and resources to individuals affected by lung disease and their family members. The Foundation, which has a head office in London and six branch offices throughout the UK, offers free membership in its 'Breathe Easy Club' to affected individuals, family members, and other caregivers. The club serves as a support and information network throughout the UK for individuals with any form of lung disease and those who care for them. Members of the Breathe Easy Club receive support and information through the 'Keep in Touch' contact service, local support groups, and a quarterly magazine entitled 'Breathe Easy.' The British Lung Foundation also provides information about all aspects of good lung health and the prevention, diagnosis, and treatment of respiratory disease through its leaflet series and 'The Lung Report.' The Foundation also has a web site on the Internet.

Relevant area(s) of interest: Sarcoidosis

- **Canadian Liver Foundation**

  Address: Canadian Liver Foundation 365 Bloor Street, Suite 200, Toronto, Ontario, M4W 3L4, Canada

  Telephone: (416) 964-493 Toll-free: (800) 563-5483

  Fax: (416) 964-0024

  Email: clf@liver.ca

  Web Site: http://www.liver.ca

  Background: The Canadian Liver Foundation (CLF) is a not-for-profit health organization committed to reducing the incidence and impact of liver disease by providing support for research and education into the causes, diagnosis, prevention and treatment of more than 100 diseases of the liver. Established in 1969, the CLF has established 30 chapters across Canada and provides information in both English and French. Some of the liver diseases discussed in brochures and medical information sheets available from CLF include gallstones, hemochromatosis, primary biliary cirrhosis, several forms of hepatitis, porphyria, fatty liver, and liver cancer. Further information is provided on liver transplantation, the effects of sodium, and management of variceal bleeding. The Foundation also produces a newsletter and maintains World Wide Web site at http://www.liver.ca.

  Relevant area(s) of interest: Sarcoidosis

- **Giant Cell Myocarditis Registry**

  Address: Giant Cell Myocarditis Registry Mayo Clinic, ATTN: Leslie T. Cooper, M.D., 200 First Street SW, Rochester, MN 55905

  Telephone: (507) 284-3680

  Fax: (507) 266-1617

  Email: cooper.leslie@mayo.edu

  Web Site: http://www.mayo.edu/cv/wwwpg_cv/research/cv_trial.htm Number gcm-ir

Background: The Giant Cell Myocarditis Study Group was established in 1994 to gather a multicenter database on Idiopathic Giant Cell Myocarditis and the related disorder Cardiac Sarcoidosis. Giant Cell Myocarditis (GCM), a rare disorder that presents with inflammation of the heart muscle, often affects young, previously healthy individuals. GCM is characterized by the progressive inability of the heart to pump blood effectively to the lungs and the rest of the body (progressive congestive heart failure) and irregularities in the rhythm of the heartbeat (arrhythmias) originating in the lower chambers of the heart (ventricular arrhythmia), resulting in potentially life-threatening complications. Cardiac Sarcoidosis, which is frequently confused with GCM due to similar symptoms and clinical findings, is chararacterized by involvement of the heart in Sarcoidosis. Sarcoidosis, a rare multisystem disorder of unknown cause, is characterized by the formation of rounded, granular, inflammatory nodules (tubercles) consisting of cells resembling those that line internal and external surfaces of the body (epithelioid tissue). The Giant Cell Myocarditis Registry conducts several clinical observational studies to better define the natural history, demographics, and effect of treatment on Giant Cell Myocarditis and Cardiac Sarcoidosis. In addition to the efforts to define the clinical spectrum of these disorders, the Registry seeks to better define the causes of Giant Cell Myocarditis in an effort to produce more effective treatments. The Registry also enables interested registry participants to network with one another, promoting understanding of the disorder and enabling affected individuals and family members to better cope with GCM. In addition, the Registry provides reprints from the peer-reviewed medical literature and bibliographies of medical journal article citations concerning Giant Cell Myocarditis and Cardiac Sarcoidosis.

- **Sarcoid Networking Association**

  Address:

  Telephone: (253) 891-688

  Fax: (253) 845-3108

  Email: sarcoidosis_netwrk@prodigy.net

  Background: The Sarcoid Networking Association (SNA) is a national not-for-profit self-help organization dedicated to providing information and support to individuals and family members affected by sarcoidosis. Sarcoidosis, a rare multisystem disorder of unknown cause, is characterized by the abnormal formation of inflammatory masses or nodules (granulomas) consisting of certain granular white blood cells (modified macrophages or epithelioid cells) in certain organs of the body.

The granulomas that are formed are thought to affect the normal structure of and, potentially, the normal functions of the affected organ(s), causing symptoms associated with the particular body system(s) in question. In individuals with sarcoidosis, such granuloma formation most commonly affects the lungs. However, in many cases, other organs may be affected. The range and severity of symptoms associated with sarcoidosis vary greatly, depending upon the specific organ(s) involved and the degree of such involvement. Established in 1992, the Sarcoid Networking Association promotes research, works to increase professional and public awareness of sarcoidosis, and provides networking services that enable affected individuals and family members to exchange information, support, and resources. The Association also engages in patient advocacy, has a directory, makes appropriate referrals, and offers a variety of materials including pamphlets, brochures, audiovisual aids, and a regular newsletter entitled 'Sarcoidosis Networking.'.

Relevant area(s) of interest: Sarcoidosis

- **Sarcoidosis Network Foundation, Inc**

Address: Sarcoidosis Network Foundation, Inc. 13337 East South Street, Suite 420, Cerritos, CA 90703

Telephone: (714) 739-139

Fax: (714) 739-1398

Background: The Sarcoidosis Network Foundation, Inc. is a nonprofit organization dedicated to supporting research into the cause, cure, and prevention of sarcoidosis; promoting education and awareness; and improving the quality of life of those affected by this disorder. Sarcoidosis, a rare multisystem disorder of unknown cause, is characterized by the abnormal formation of inflammatory masses or nodules (granulomas) consisting of certain granular white blood cells (modified macrophages or epithelioid cells) in certain organs of the body. The granulomas that are formed are thought to affect the normal structure of and, potentially, the normal functions of the affected organ(s), causing symptoms associated with the particular body system(s) in question. In individuals with sarcoidosis, such granuloma formation most commonly affects the lungs. However, in many cases, other organs may be affected. The range and severity of symptoms associated with sarcoidosis vary greatly, depending upon the specific organ(s) involved and the degree of such involvement. Established in 1992, the Sarcoidosis Network Foundation provides educational materials about sarcoidosis including a quarterly newsletter entitled

'R.E.A.C.H.'; offers monthly support groups for affected individuals, family members, and caregivers; provides disability, counseling, and physician referrals; and offers patient networking services to enable affected individuals and family members to share their experiences with others.

Relevant area(s) of interest: Sarcoid of Boeck, Sarcoidosis, Schaumann's Disease

- **Sarcoidosis Online Sites: A Comprehensive Source for SarcoidosisInformation on the Internet**

  Address: Sarcoidosis Online Sites: A Comprehensive Source for Sarcoidosis Information on the Internet

  Email: JaysJob@aol.com

  Web Site: http://members.aol.com/jaysjob/sarcoid/sos1.html Number TOP

  Background: Sarcoidosis Online Sites: A Comprehensive Source for Sarcoidosis Information on the Internet is a web site dedicated to educating individuals with sarcoidosis, family members, and friends; helping in the search for treatments and cure for sarcoidosis; providing online networking opportunities for those affected by the disorder; and increasing awareness of sarcoidosis and bringing the disorder to the forefront of the medical, research, and general communities. Sarcoidosis, a rare multisystem disorder of unknown cause, is characterized by the abnormal formation of inflammatory masses or nodules (granulomas) consisting of certain granular white blood cells (modified macrophages or epithelioid cells) in certain organs of the body. The granulomas that are formed are thought to affect the normal structure of and, potentially, the normal functions of the affected organ(s), causing symptoms associated with the particular body system(s) in question. In individuals with sarcoidosis, such granuloma formation most commonly affects the lungs. However, in many cases, other organs may be affected. The range and severity of symptoms associated with sarcoidosis vary greatly, depending upon the specific organ(s) involved and the degree of such involvement. Sarcoidosis Online Sites (S.O.S.) provides descriptions of and dynamic linkage to sarcoidosis related web pages under several categories including What is Sarcoidosis?, Diagnostic Testing, Medication Information, Hospital Resources, Organizations, University Resources, and Chronic Pain. The site also provides online networking opportunities through its guestbook and produces and maintains the 'NSRC Sarcoidosis Community Newsletter,' a monthly online newsletter.

Relevant area(s) of interest: Sarcoid of Boeck, Sarcoidosis, Schaumann's Disease

- **Sarcoidosis Research Institute**

  Address: Sarcoidosis Research Institute 3475 Central Avenue, Memphis, TN 38111

  Telephone: (901) 766-6951

  Fax: (901) 774-7294

  Email: soskelnt@netten.net

  Web Site: http://www.netten.net/~soskelnt/

  Background: The Sarcoidosis Research Institute is a national not-for-profit organization established in 1991. The Institute is dedicated to providing up-to-date information to individuals with sarcoidosis and conducting forums for affected individuals and their families. Sarcoidosis, a rare multisystem disorder of unknown cause, is characterized by the abnormal formation of inflammatory masses or nodules (granulomas) consisting of certain granular white blood cells (modified macrophages or epithelioid cells) in certain organs of the body. The granulomas that are formed are thought to affect the normal structure of and, potentially, the normal functions of the affected organ(s), causing symptoms associated with the particular body system(s) in question. In individuals with sarcoidosis, such granuloma formation most commonly affects the lungs. However, in many cases, other organs may be affected. The range and severity of symptoms associated with sarcoidosis vary greatly, depending upon the specific organ(s) involved and the degree of such involvement. The Sarcoidosis Research Institute is also dedicated to increasing public awareness of sarcoidosis and channeling appropriate information to the medical community. Educational materials produced by the Sarcoidosis Research Institute include a brochure entitled 'Answers to Your Questions about Sarcoidosis' and a video called 'Sarcoidosis: An Overview.'.

  Relevant area(s) of interest: Sarcoid of Boeck, Sarcoidosis, Schaumann's Disease

- **Second Wind Lung Transplant Association, Inc**

  Address: Second Wind Lung Transplant Association, Inc. 300 South Duncan Avenue, Suite 227, Clearwater, FL 33755

  Telephone: (212) 668-1000 Toll-free: (888) 222-2690

  Fax: (727) 442- 9762

Email: secondwind@netzero.net

Web Site: http://www.2ndwind.org

Background: Second Wind Lung Transplant Association, Inc. is a not-for-profit organization dedicated to improving the quality of life for lung transplant recipients, lung surgery candidates, people with related pulmonary concerns, and their families. The Association provides support, advocacy, education, information, and guidance through a spirit of service, 'adding years to their lives and life to their years.' Established in 1995 by a group of lung transplant recipients, candidates, and their families, Second Wind has quarterly support group meetings to provide educational programs (e.g., on nutrition, effects of medications and exercise, physical therapy) for both lung transplant candidates and recipients; to share experiences; and to enjoy social activities. Second Wind also is developing a directory of candidates and lung transplant recipients to provide networking opportunities; is establishing a mentor program to offer fellowship to affected individuals and families during the transplant experience; and is planning to establish low-cost Lung Transplant Housing near transplant hospitals for use by candidate and recipient transplant affected individuals and their support person. In addition, the organization provides educational programs; seeks to increase Organ Donor Awareness; and provides a quarterly newsletter entitled 'AirWays' to their members. The Second Wind Lung Transplant Association also has a web site on the Internet that provides information to individuals who seek information on lung transplantation. The site also provides linkage to information on certain specific pulmonary disorders; describes Second Wind's mentoring program; and provides information concerning financing lung transplantation. Such information includes listings of organizations that may provide advocacy, assistance with fund-raising, financial grants, and/or medication or pharmaceutical payment assistance grants or programs.

Relevant area(s) of interest: Sarcoidosis

Finding More Associations

There are a number of directories that list additional medical associations that you may find useful. While not all of these directories will provide different information than what is listed above, by consulting all of them, you will have nearly exhausted all sources for patient associations.

The National Health Information Center (NHIC)

The National Health Information Center (NHIC) offers a free referral service to help people find organizations that provide information about sarcoidosis. For more information, see the NHIC's Web site at **http://www.health.gov/NHIC/** or contact an information specialist by calling 1-800-336-4797.

DIRLINE

A comprehensive source of information on associations is the DIRLINE database maintained by the National Library of Medicine. The database comprises some 10,000 records of organizations, research centers, and government institutes and associations which primarily focus on health and biomedicine. DIRLINE is available via the Internet at the following Web site: **http://dirline.nlm.nih.gov/**. Simply type in "sarcoidosis" (or a synonym) or the name of a topic, and the site will list information contained in the database on all relevant organizations.

The Combined Health Information Database

Another comprehensive source of information on healthcare associations is the Combined Health Information Database. Using the "Detailed Search" option, you will need to limit your search to "Organizations" and "sarcoidosis". Type the following hyperlink into your Web browser: **http://chid.nih.gov/detail/detail.html**. To find associations, use the drop boxes at the bottom of the search page where "You may refine your search by." For publication date, select "All Years." Then, select your preferred language and the format option "Organization Resource Sheet." By making these selections and typing in "sarcoidosis" (or synonyms) into the "For these words:" box, you will only receive results on organizations dealing with sarcoidosis. You should check back periodically with this database since it is updated every 3 months.

The National Organization for Rare Disorders, Inc.

The National Organization for Rare Disorders, Inc. has prepared a Web site that provides, at no charge, lists of associations organized by specific diseases. You can access this database at the following Web site: **http://www.rarediseases.org/cgi-bin/nord/searchpage**. Select the option called "Organizational Database (ODB)" and type "sarcoidosis" (or a synonym) in the search box.

Online Support Groups

In addition to support groups, commercial Internet service providers offer forums and chat rooms for people with different illnesses and conditions. WebMD®, for example, offers such a service at their Web site: **http://boards.webmd.com/roundtable**. These online self-help communities can help you connect with a network of people whose concerns are similar to yours. Online support groups are places where people can talk informally. If you read about a novel approach, consult with your doctor or other healthcare providers, as the treatments or discoveries you hear about may not be scientifically proven to be safe and effective.

- **Sarcoidosis Online Sites**
  http://www.sarcoidosisonlinesites.com/

- **Sarcoidosis Support Group**
  http://pobox.upenn.edu/~jmclauri/supp.html

- **Sarcoidosis Worldwide Support Group**
  http://www.geocities.com/HotSprings/Spa/9139/

Finding Doctors

One of the most important aspects of your treatment will be the relationship between you and your doctor or specialist. All patients with sarcoidosis must go through the process of selecting a physician. While this process will vary from person to person, the Agency for Healthcare Research and Quality makes a number of suggestions, including the following:[11]

- If you are in a managed care plan, check the plan's list of doctors first.

- Ask doctors or other health professionals who work with doctors, such as hospital nurses, for referrals.

- Call a hospital's doctor referral service, but keep in mind that these services usually refer you to doctors on staff at that particular hospital.

---

[11] This section is adapted from the AHRQ: www.ahrq.gov/consumer/qntascii/qntdr.htm.

The services do not have information on the quality of care that these doctors provide.

- Some local medical societies offer lists of member doctors. Again, these lists do not have information on the quality of care that these doctors provide.

Additional steps you can take to locate doctors include the following:

- Check with the associations listed earlier in this chapter.

- Information on doctors in some states is available on the Internet at **http://www.docboard.org**. This Web site is run by "Administrators in Medicine," a group of state medical board directors.

- The American Board of Medical Specialties can tell you if your doctor is board certified. "Certified" means that the doctor has completed a training program in a specialty and has passed an exam, or "board," to assess his or her knowledge, skills, and experience to provide quality patient care in that specialty. Primary care doctors may also be certified as specialists. The AMBS Web site is located at **http://www.abms.org/newsearch.asp**.[12] You can also contact the ABMS by phone at 1-866-ASK-ABMS.

- You can call the American Medical Association (AMA) at 800-665-2882 for information on training, specialties, and board certification for many licensed doctors in the United States. This information also can be found in "Physician Select" at the AMA's Web site: **http://www.ama-assn.org/aps/amahg.htm**.

If the previous sources did not meet your needs, you may want to log on to the Web site of the National Organization for Rare Disorders (NORD) at **http://www.rarediseases.org/**. NORD maintains a database of doctors with expertise in various rare diseases. The Metabolic Information Network (MIN), 800-945-2188, also maintains a database of physicians with expertise in various metabolic diseases.

---

[12] While board certification is a good measure of a doctor's knowledge, it is possible to receive quality care from doctors who are not board certified.

Selecting Your Doctor[13]

When you have compiled a list of prospective doctors, call each of their offices. First, ask if the doctor accepts your health insurance plan and if he or she is taking new patients. If the doctor is not covered by your plan, ask yourself if you are prepared to pay the extra costs. The next step is to schedule a visit with your chosen physician. During the first visit you will have the opportunity to evaluate your doctor and to find out if you feel comfortable with him or her. Ask yourself, did the doctor:

- Give me a chance to ask questions about sarcoidosis?

- Really listen to my questions?

- Answer in terms I understood?

- Show respect for me?

- Ask me questions?

- Make me feel comfortable?

- Address the health problem(s) I came with?

- Ask me my preferences about different kinds of treatments for sarcoidosis?

- Spend enough time with me?

Trust your instincts when deciding if the doctor is right for you. But remember, it might take time for the relationship to develop. It takes more than one visit for you and your doctor to get to know each other.

Working with Your Doctor[14]

Research has shown that patients who have good relationships with their doctors tend to be more satisfied with their care and have better results. Here are some tips to help you and your doctor become partners:

- You know important things about your symptoms and your health history. Tell your doctor what you think he or she needs to know.

---

[13] This section has been adapted from the AHRQ:
www.ahrq.gov/consumer/qntascii/qntdr.htm.
[14] This section has been adapted from the AHRQ:
www.ahrq.gov/consumer/qntascii/qntdr.htm.

- It is important to tell your doctor personal information, even if it makes you feel embarrassed or uncomfortable.

- Bring a "health history" list with you (and keep it up to date).

- Always bring any medications you are currently taking with you to the appointment, or you can bring a list of your medications including dosage and frequency information. Talk about any allergies or reactions you have had to your medications.

- Tell your doctor about any natural or alternative medicines you are taking.

- Bring other medical information, such as x-ray films, test results, and medical records.

- Ask questions. If you don't, your doctor will assume that you understood everything that was said.

- Write down your questions before your visit. List the most important ones first to make sure that they are addressed.

- Consider bringing a friend with you to the appointment to help you ask questions. This person can also help you understand and/or remember the answers.

- Ask your doctor to draw pictures if you think that this would help you understand.

- Take notes. Some doctors do not mind if you bring a tape recorder to help you remember things, but always ask first.

- Let your doctor know if you need more time. If there is not time that day, perhaps you can speak to a nurse or physician assistant on staff or schedule a telephone appointment.

- Take information home. Ask for written instructions. Your doctor may also have brochures and audio and videotapes that can help you.

- After leaving the doctor's office, take responsibility for your care. If you have questions, call. If your symptoms get worse or if you have problems with your medication, call. If you had tests and do not hear from your doctor, call for your test results. If your doctor recommended that you have certain tests, schedule an appointment to get them done. If your doctor said you should see an additional specialist, make an appointment.

By following these steps, you will enhance the relationship you will have with your physician.

Broader Health-Related Resources

In addition to the references above, the NIH has set up guidance Web sites that can help patients find healthcare professionals. These include:[15]

- Caregivers:
  http://www.nlm.nih.gov/medlineplus/caregivers.html

- Choosing a Doctor or Healthcare Service:
  http://www.nlm.nih.gov/medlineplus/choosingadoctororhealthcareserv ice.html

- Hospitals and Health Facilities:
  http://www.nlm.nih.gov/medlineplus/healthfacilities.html

Vocabulary Builder

The following vocabulary builder provides definitions of words used in this chapter that have not been defined in previous chapters:

Anaphylaxis: An acute hypersensitivity reaction due to exposure to a previously encountered antigen. The reaction may include rapidly progressing urticaria, respiratory distress, vascular collapse, systemic shock, and death. [NIH]

Arrhythmia: An irregular heartbeat. [NIH]

Autoimmunity: Process whereby the immune system reacts against the body's own tissues. Autoimmunity may produce or be caused by autoimmune diseases. [NIH]

Biliary: Pertaining to the bile, to the bile ducts, or to the gallbladder. [EU]

Bronchitis: Inflammation of one or more bronchi. [EU]

Cardiac: Pertaining to the heart. [EU]

Cirrhosis: Liver disease characterized pathologically by loss of the normal microscopic lobular architecture, with fibrosis and nodular regeneration. The term is sometimes used to refer to chronic interstitial inflammation of any organ. [EU]

Emphysema: Chronic lung disease in which there is permanent destruction of alveoli. [NIH]

---

[15] You can access this information at:
http://www.nlm.nih.gov/medlineplus/healthsystem.html.

Epidemiological: Relating to, or involving epidemiology. [EU]

Heartbeat: One complete contraction of the heart. [NIH]

Hepatitis: Inflammation of the liver. [EU]

Idiopathic: Results from an unknown cause. [NIH]

Myocarditis: Inflammation of the myocardium; inflammation of the muscular walls of the heart. [EU]

Porphyria: A pathological state in man and some lower animals that is often due to genetic factors, is characterized by abnormalities of porphyrin metabolism, and results in the excretion of large quantities of porphyrins in the urine and in extreme sensitivity to light. [EU]

Rhinitis: Inflammation of the mucous membrane of the nose. [EU]

Spectrum: A charted band of wavelengths of electromagnetic vibrations obtained by refraction and diffraction. By extension, a measurable range of activity, such as the range of bacteria affected by an antibiotic (antibacterial s.) or the complete range of manifestations of a disease. [EU]

Transplantation: The grafting of tissues taken from the patient's own body or from another. [EU]

CHAPTER 3. CLINICAL TRIALS AND SARCOIDOSIS

Overview

Very few medical conditions have a single treatment. The basic treatment guidelines that your physician has discussed with you, or those that you have found using the techniques discussed in Chapter 1, may provide you with all that you will require. For some patients, current treatments can be enhanced with new or innovative techniques currently under investigation. In this chapter, we will describe how clinical trials work and show you how to keep informed of trials concerning sarcoidosis.

What Is a Clinical Trial?[16]

Clinical trials involve the participation of people in medical research. Most medical research begins with studies in test tubes and on animals. Treatments that show promise in these early studies may then be tried with people. The only sure way to find out whether a new treatment is safe, effective, and better than other treatments for sarcoidosis is to try it on patients in a clinical trial.

---

[16] The discussion in this chapter has been adapted from the NIH and the NEI: www.nei.nih.gov/netrials/ctivr.htm.

What Kinds of Clinical Trials Are There?

Clinical trials are carried out in three phases:

- **Phase I.** Researchers first conduct Phase I trials with small numbers of patients and healthy volunteers. If the new treatment is a medication, researchers also try to determine how much of it can be given safely.

- **Phase II.** Researchers conduct Phase II trials in small numbers of patients to find out the effect of a new treatment on sarcoidosis.

- **Phase III.** Finally, researchers conduct Phase III trials to find out how new treatments for sarcoidosis compare with standard treatments already being used. Phase III trials also help to determine if new treatments have any side effects. These trials--which may involve hundreds, perhaps thousands, of people--can also compare new treatments with no treatment.

How Is a Clinical Trial Conducted?

Various organizations support clinical trials at medical centers, hospitals, universities, and doctors' offices across the United States. The "principal investigator" is the researcher in charge of the study at each facility participating in the clinical trial. Most clinical trial researchers are medical doctors, academic researchers, and specialists. The "clinic coordinator" knows all about how the study works and makes all the arrangements for your visits.

All doctors and researchers who take part in the study on sarcoidosis carefully follow a detailed treatment plan called a protocol. This plan fully explains how the doctors will treat you in the study. The "protocol" ensures that all patients are treated in the same way, no matter where they receive care.

Clinical trials are controlled. This means that researchers compare the effects of the new treatment with those of the standard treatment. In some cases, when no standard treatment exists, the new treatment is compared with no treatment. Patients who receive the new treatment are in the treatment group. Patients who receive a standard treatment or no treatment are in the "control" group. In some clinical trials, patients in the treatment group get a new medication while those in the control group get a placebo. A placebo is a harmless substance, a "dummy" pill, that has no effect on sarcoidosis. In other clinical trials, where a new surgery or device (not a medicine) is being tested, patients in the control group may receive a "sham treatment." This treatment, like a placebo, has no effect on sarcoidosis and does not harm patients.

Researchers assign patients "randomly" to the treatment or control group. This is like flipping a coin to decide which patients are in each group. If you choose to participate in a clinical trial, you will not know which group you will be appointed to. The chance of any patient getting the new treatment is about 50 percent. You cannot request to receive the new treatment instead of the placebo or sham treatment. Often, you will not know until the study is over whether you have been in the treatment group or the control group. This is called a "masked" study. In some trials, neither doctors nor patients know who is getting which treatment. This is called a "double masked" study. These types of trials help to ensure that the perceptions of the patients or doctors will not affect the study results.

Natural History Studies

Unlike clinical trials in which patient volunteers may receive new treatments, natural history studies provide important information to researchers on how sarcoidosis develops over time. A natural history study follows patient volunteers to see how factors such as age, sex, race, or family history might make some people more or less at risk for sarcoidosis. A natural history study may also tell researchers if diet, lifestyle, or occupation affects how a disease or disorder develops and progresses. Results from these studies provide information that helps answer questions such as: How fast will a disease or disorder usually progress? How bad will the condition become? Will treatment be needed?

What Is Expected of Patients in a Clinical Trial?

Not everyone can take part in a clinical trial for a specific disease or disorder. Each study enrolls patients with certain features or eligibility criteria. These criteria may include the type and stage of disease or disorder, as well as, the age and previous treatment history of the patient. You or your doctor can contact the sponsoring organization to find out more about specific clinical trials and their eligibility criteria. If you are interested in joining a clinical trial, your doctor must contact one of the trial's investigators and provide details about your diagnosis and medical history.

If you participate in a clinical trial, you may be required to have a number of medical tests. You may also need to take medications and/or undergo surgery. Depending upon the treatment and the examination procedure, you may be required to receive inpatient hospital care. Or, you may have to return to the medical facility for follow-up examinations. These exams help find out how well the treatment is working. Follow-up studies can take months or years. However, the success of the clinical trial often depends on learning what happens to patients over a long period of time. Only patients who continue to return for follow-up examinations can provide this important long-term information.

Recent Trials on Sarcoidosis

The National Institutes of Health and other organizations sponsor trials on various diseases and disorders. Because funding for research goes to the medical areas that show promising research opportunities, it is not possible for the NIH or others to sponsor clinical trials for every disease and disorder at all times. The following lists recent trials dedicated to sarcoidosis.[17] If the trial listed by the NIH is still recruiting, you may be eligible. If it is no longer recruiting or has been completed, then you can contact the sponsors to learn more about the study and, if published, the results. Further information on the trial is available at the Web site indicated. Please note that some trials may no longer be recruiting patients or are otherwise closed. Before contacting sponsors of a clinical trial, consult with your physician who can help you determine if you might benefit from participation.

- **Evaluation and Follow-up of Patients with Cryptococcosis**

  Condition(s): Cryptococcosis; Lymphopenia

  Study Status: This study is currently recruiting patients.

  Sponsor(s): National Institute of Allergy and Infectious Diseases (NIAID)

  Purpose - Excerpt: This 5-year study will follow the course of disease in previously healthy patients with cryptococcosis who developed the disease for no identifiable reason. Individuals with a positive culture of Cryptococcus neoformans 18 years of age and older without HIV infection or other condition predisposing to cryptococcosis (such as high-dose corticosteroid therapy, sarcoidosis, or a blood cancer) may be eligible for this study. Candidates who test positive for HIV infection may not participate. Participants will have a physical examination, medical history, routine blood tests and assessment of disease activity upon entering the study. Patients who may have active cryptococcosis will also have a lumbar puncture (spinal tap) and additional blood tests. Following the initial evaluation, patients receiving treatment for

---

[17] These are listed at www.ClinicalTrials.gov.

cryptococcosis will come to the NIH Clinical Center as needed to manage their disease, typically no less than every 3 months. Other patients will be seen every 6 to 12 months. The visits will include a medical history, physical examination, and blood and urine tests.

Study Type: Observational

Contact(s): Maryland; National Institute of Allergy and Infectious Diseases (NIAID), 9000 Rockville Pike Bethesda, Maryland, 20892, United States; Recruiting; Patient Recruitment and Public Liaison Office 1-800-411-1222 prpl@mail.cc.nih.gov; TTY 1-866-411-1010

Web Site: http://clinicaltrials.gov/ct/gui/c/w2r/show/NCT00001352

- **Role of Genetic Factors in the Development of Lung Disease**

  Condition(s): Alpha 1 Antitrypsin Deficiency; Cystic Fibrosis; Lung Disease; Obstructive Lung Disease; Sarcoidosis

  Study Status: This study is currently recruiting patients.

  Sponsor(s): National Heart, Lung, and Blood Institute (NHLBI)

  Purpose - Excerpt: This study is designed to evaluate the genetics involved in the development of lung disease by surveying genes involved in the process of breathing and examining the genes in lung cells of patients with lung disease. The study will focus on defining the distribution of abnormal genes responsible for processes directly involved in different diseases affecting the lungs of patients and healthy volunteers.

  Study Type: Observational

  Contact(s): Maryland; National Heart, Lung and Blood Institute (NHLBI), 9000 Rockville Pike Bethesda, Maryland, 20892, United States; Recruiting; Patient Recruitment and Public Liaison Office 1-800-411-1222 prpl@mail.cc.nih.gov; TTY 1-866-411-1010

  Web Site: http://clinicaltrials.gov/ct/gui/c/w2r/show/NCT00001532

- **Sarcoid Genetic Analysis (SAGA)**

  Condition(s): Lung Diseases; Sarcoidosis

  Study Status: This study is currently recruiting patients.

  Sponsor(s): National Heart, Lung, and Blood Institute (NHLBI)

  Purpose - Excerpt: To identify sarcoidosis susceptibility genes and to determine how these genes and environmental risk factors interact to cause sarcoidosis.

  Contact(s): see Web site below

Web Site: http://clinicaltrials.gov/ct/gui/c/w2r/show/NCT00005542

- **Treatment of Pulmonary Sarcoidosis with Pentoxifylline**

  Condition(s): Pulmonary Sarcoidosis

  Study Status: This study is currently recruiting patients.

  Sponsor(s): National Heart, Lung, and Blood Institute (NHLBI)

  Purpose - Excerpt: Sarcoidosis is a disease most commonly affecting the lungs, but it can also involve lymph nodes, skin, liver, spleen, eyes, bones, and glands. The cause of the disease is unknown. When it occurs it can produce an inflammatory reaction leading to irreversible organ damage and disability. In sarcoidosis granulomas can form in various organs (primarily lung) which can lead to its dysfunction. Granuloma is formed by clusters of inflammatory cells. The formation of these granulomas is influenced by the release of a substance called TNF-alpha (tumor necrosis factor alpha) which is found in some white blood cells. A drug known as pentoxifylline (POF) is known to markedly reduce the release of TNF-alpha. The standard medical treatment for sarcoidosis is steroid therapy. However, steroid therapy is associated with significant side effects and often must be stopped. Unfortunately, some of these patients can relapse when the steroid therapy is discontinued. Because of this, researchers are interested in finding alternative therapies for the treatment of sarcoidosis. This study will evaluate the effectiveness of giving POF to patients with sarcoidosis currently taking steroids. Researchers will compare the results between patients taking steroids with pentoxifylline and those patients taking steroids alone.

  Phase(s): Phase II

  Study Type: Interventional

  Contact(s): Maryland; National Heart, Lung and Blood Institute (NHLBI), 9000 Rockville Pike Bethesda, Maryland, 20892, United States; Recruiting; Patient Recruitment and Public Liaison Office 1-800-411-1222 prpl@mail.cc.nih.gov; TTY 1-866-411-1010

  Web Site: http://clinicaltrials.gov/ct/gui/c/w2r/show/NCT00001877

- **Case Control Epidemiologic Study of Sarcoidosis (ACCESS)**

  Condition(s): Lung Diseases; Sarcoidosis

  Study Status: This study is no longer recruiting patients.

  Sponsor(s): National Heart, Lung, and Blood Institute (NHLBI)

  Purpose - Excerpt: To test specific hypotheses concerning environmental, occupational, lifestyle, and other risk factors for sarcoidosis. Also, to examine the familial aggregation of sarcoidosis and to test genetic hypotheses concerning its etiology. Finally, to describe the natural history of sarcoidosis, particularly in African-Americans who appear to be disproportionately affected, and to implement a system for storing biological specimens including blood cells, plasma, and serum.

Study Type: Epidemiology

Contact(s): see Web site below

Web Site: http://clinicaltrials.gov/ct/gui/c/w2r/show/NCT00005276

- **Diffuse Fibrotic Lung Disease**

  Condition(s): Lung Diseases; Pulmonary Fibrosis; Sarcoidosis

  Study Status: This study is completed.

  Sponsor(s): National Heart, Lung, and Blood Institute (NHLBI)

  Purpose - Excerpt: To determine the effects of cyclophosphamide compared with prednisone, dapsone, or high-dose intermittent 'pulse' therapy with methylprednisolone in patients with idiopathic pulmonary fibrosis. Also, to evaluate the use of intermittent, short-term, high-dose intravenous corticosteroids in patients with sarcoidosis. There were actually four separate clinical trials.

  Phase(s): Phase II

  Study Type: Treatment

  Contact(s): Crystal, Ronald G. Bethesda, Maryland, United States . Study chairs or principal investigators: Crystal, Ronald G., Study Chair; Pulmonary Branch, NHLBI Bethesda, Maryland, United States

  Web Site: http://clinicaltrials.gov/ct/gui/c/w2r/show/NCT00000596

- **Genetic Epidemiology of Sarcoidosis**

  Condition(s): Lung Diseases; Sarcoidosis

  Study Status: This study is completed.

  Sponsor(s): National Heart, Lung, and Blood Institute (NHLBI)

  Purpose - Excerpt: To determine if hereditary susceptibility predisposes African Americans to sarcoidosis and to identify sarcoidosis susceptibility genes in African Americans.

  Study Type: Epidemiology

  Contact(s): see Web site below

  Web Site: http://clinicaltrials.gov/ct/gui/c/w2r/show/NCT00005531

Benefits and Risks[18]

What Are the Benefits of Participating in a Clinical Trial?

If you are interested in a clinical trial, it is important to realize that your participation can bring many benefits to you and society at large:

- A new treatment could be more effective than the current treatment for sarcoidosis. Although only half of the participants in a clinical trial receive the experimental treatment, if the new treatment is proved to be more effective and safer than the current treatment, then those patients who did not receive the new treatment during the clinical trial may be among the first to benefit from it when the study is over.

- If the treatment is effective, then it may improve health or prevent diseases or disorders.

- Clinical trial patients receive the highest quality of medical care. Experts watch them closely during the study and may continue to follow them after the study is over.

- People who take part in trials contribute to scientific discoveries that may help other people with sarcoidosis. In cases where certain diseases or disorders run in families, your participation may lead to better care or prevention for your family members.

The Informed Consent

Once you agree to take part in a clinical trial, you will be asked to sign an "informed consent." This document explains a clinical trial's risks and benefits, the researcher's expectations of you, and your rights as a patient.

What Are the Risks?

Clinical trials may involve risks as well as benefits. Whether or not a new treatment will work cannot be known ahead of time. There is always a chance that a new treatment may not work better than a standard treatment. There is also the possibility that it may be harmful. The treatment you receive may cause side effects that are serious enough to require medical attention.

---

[18] This section has been adapted from ClinicalTrials.gov, a service of the National Institutes of Health:
http://www.clinicaltrials.gov/ct/gui/c/a1r/info/whatis?JServSessionIdzone_ct=9jmun6f291.

How Is Patient Safety Protected?

Clinical trials can raise fears of the unknown. Understanding the safeguards that protect patients can ease some of these fears. Before a clinical trial begins, researchers must get approval from their hospital's Institutional Review Board (IRB), an advisory group that makes sure a clinical trial is designed to protect patient safety. During a clinical trial, doctors will closely watch you to see if the treatment is working and if you are experiencing any side effects. All the results are carefully recorded and reviewed. In many cases, experts from the Data and Safety Monitoring Committee carefully monitor each clinical trial and can recommend that a study be stopped at any time. You will only be asked to take part in a clinical trial as a volunteer giving informed consent.

What Are a Patient's Rights in a Clinical Trial?

If you are eligible for a clinical trial, you will be given information to help you decide whether or not you want to participate. As a patient, you have the right to:

- Information on all known risks and benefits of the treatments in the study.

- Know how the researchers plan to carry out the study, for how long, and where.

- Know what is expected of you.

- Know any costs involved for you or your insurance provider.

- Know before any of your medical or personal information is shared with other researchers involved in the clinical trial.

- Talk openly with doctors and ask any questions.

After you join a clinical trial, you have the right to:

- Leave the study at any time. Participation is strictly voluntary. However, you should not enroll if you do not plan to complete the study.

- Receive any new information about the new treatment.

- Continue to ask questions and get answers.

- Maintain your privacy. Your name will not appear in any reports based on the study.

- Know whether you participated in the treatment group or the control group (once the study has been completed).

What about Costs?

In some clinical trials, the research facility pays for treatment costs and other associated expenses. You or your insurance provider may have to pay for costs that are considered standard care. These things may include inpatient hospital care, laboratory and other tests, and medical procedures. You also may need to pay for travel between your home and the clinic. You should find out about costs before committing to participation in the trial. If you have health insurance, find out exactly what it will cover. If you don't have health insurance, or if your insurance company will not cover your costs, talk to the clinic staff about other options for covering the cost of your care.

What Should You Ask before Deciding to Join a Clinical Trial?

Questions you should ask when thinking about joining a clinical trial include the following:

- What is the purpose of the clinical trial?
- What are the standard treatments for sarcoidosis? Why do researchers think the new treatment may be better? What is likely to happen to me with or without the new treatment?
- What tests and treatments will I need? Will I need surgery? Medication? Hospitalization?
- How long will the treatment last? How often will I have to come back for follow-up exams?
- What are the treatment's possible benefits to my condition? What are the short- and long-term risks? What are the possible side effects?
- Will the treatment be uncomfortable? Will it make me feel sick? If so, for how long?
- How will my health be monitored?
- Where will I need to go for the clinical trial? How will I get there?
- How much will it cost to be in the study? What costs are covered by the study? How much will my health insurance cover?
- Will I be able to see my own doctor? Who will be in charge of my care?

- Will taking part in the study affect my daily life? Do I have time to participate?

- How do I feel about taking part in a clinical trial? Are there family members or friends who may benefit from my contributions to new medical knowledge?

Keeping Current on Clinical Trials

Various government agencies maintain databases on trials. The U.S. National Institutes of Health, through the National Library of Medicine, has developed ClinicalTrials.gov to provide patients, family members, and physicians with current information about clinical research across the broadest number of diseases and conditions.

The site was launched in February 2000 and currently contains approximately 5,700 clinical studies in over 59,000 locations worldwide, with most studies being conducted in the United States. ClinicalTrials.gov receives about 2 million hits per month and hosts approximately 5,400 visitors daily. To access this database, simply go to their Web site (**www.clinicaltrials.gov**) and search by "sarcoidosis" (or synonyms).

While ClinicalTrials.gov is the most comprehensive listing of NIH-supported clinical trials available, not all trials are in the database. The database is updated regularly, so clinical trials are continually being added. The following is a list of specialty databases affiliated with the National Institutes of Health that offer additional information on trials:

- For clinical studies at the Warren Grant Magnuson Clinical Center located in Bethesda, Maryland, visit their Web site: **http://clinicalstudies.info.nih.gov/**

- For clinical studies conducted at the Bayview Campus in Baltimore, Maryland, visit their Web site: **http://www.jhbmc.jhu.edu/studies/index.html**

- For heart, lung and blood trials, visit the Web page of the National Heart, Lung and Blood Institute: **http://www.nhlbi.nih.gov/studies/index.htm**

General References

The following references describe clinical trials and experimental medical research. They have been selected to ensure that they are likely to be available from your local or online bookseller or university medical library. These references are usually written for healthcare professionals, so you may consider consulting with a librarian or bookseller who might recommend a particular reference. The following includes some of the most readily available references (sorted alphabetically by title; hyperlinks provide rankings, information and reviews at Amazon.com):

- **A Guide to Patient Recruitment : Today's Best Practices & Proven Strategies** by Diana L. Anderson; Paperback - 350 pages (2001), CenterWatch, Inc.; ISBN: 1930624115; http://www.amazon.com/exec/obidos/ASIN/1930624115/icongroupinterna

- **A Step-By-Step Guide to Clinical Trials** by Marilyn Mulay, R.N., M.S., OCN; Spiral-bound - 143 pages Spiral edition (2001), Jones & Bartlett Pub; ISBN: 0763715697; http://www.amazon.com/exec/obidos/ASIN/0763715697/icongroupinterna

- **The CenterWatch Directory of Drugs in Clinical Trials** by CenterWatch; Paperback - 656 pages (2000), CenterWatch, Inc.; ISBN: 0967302935; http://www.amazon.com/exec/obidos/ASIN/0967302935/icongroupinterna

- **The Complete Guide to Informed Consent in Clinical Trials** by Terry Hartnett (Editor); Paperback - 164 pages (2000), PharmSource Information Services, Inc.; ISBN: 0970153309; http://www.amazon.com/exec/obidos/ASIN/0970153309/icongroupinterna

- **Dictionary for Clinical Trials** by Simon Day; Paperback - 228 pages (1999), John Wiley & Sons; ISBN: 0471985961; http://www.amazon.com/exec/obidos/ASIN/0471985961/icongroupinterna

- **Extending Medicare Reimbursement in Clinical Trials** by Institute of Medicine Staff (Editor), et al; Paperback 1st edition (2000), National Academy Press; ISBN: 0309068886; http://www.amazon.com/exec/obidos/ASIN/0309068886/icongroupinterna

- **Handbook of Clinical Trials** by Marcus Flather (Editor); Paperback (2001), Remedica Pub Ltd; ISBN: 1901346293; http://www.amazon.com/exec/obidos/ASIN/1901346293/icongroupinterna

Vocabulary Builder

The following vocabulary builder gives definitions of words used in this chapter that have not been defined in previous chapters:

Cryptococcosis: Infection with a fungus of the species cryptococcus neoformans. [NIH]

Cryptococcus: A mitosporic Tremellales fungal genus whose species usually have a capsule and do not form pseudomycellium. Teleomorphs include Filobasidiella and Fidobasidium. [NIH]

Intravenous: Within a vein or veins. [EU]

Lumbar: Pertaining to the loins, the part of the back between the thorax and the pelvis. [EU]

Lymphopenia: Reduction in the number of lymphocytes. [NIH]

Necrosis: The sum of the morphological changes indicative of cell death and caused by the progressive degradative action of enzymes; it may affect groups of cells or part of a structure or an organ. [EU]

Pentoxifylline: A methylxanthine derivative that inhibits phosphodiesterase and affects blood rheology. It improves blood flow by increasing erythrocyte and leukocyte flexibility. It also inhibits platelet aggregation. Pentoxifylline modulates immunologic activity by stimulating cytokine production. [NIH]

PART II: ADDITIONAL RESOURCES AND ADVANCED MATERIAL

ABOUT PART II

In Part II, we introduce you to additional resources and advanced research on sarcoidosis. All too often, patients who conduct their own research are overwhelmed by the difficulty in finding and organizing information. The purpose of the following chapters is to provide you an organized and structured format to help you find additional information resources on sarcoidosis. In Part II, as in Part I, our objective is not to interpret the latest advances on sarcoidosis or render an opinion. Rather, our goal is to give you access to original research and to increase your awareness of sources you may not have already considered. In this way, you will come across the advanced materials often referred to in pamphlets, books, or other general works. Once again, some of this material is technical in nature, so consultation with a professional familiar with sarcoidosis is suggested.

Chapter 4. Studies on Sarcoidosis

Overview

Every year, academic studies are published on sarcoidosis or related conditions. Broadly speaking, there are two types of studies. The first are peer reviewed. Generally, the content of these studies has been reviewed by scientists or physicians. Peer-reviewed studies are typically published in scientific journals and are usually available at medical libraries. The second type of studies is non-peer reviewed. These works include summary articles that do not use or report scientific results. These often appear in the popular press, newsletters, or similar periodicals.

In this chapter, we will show you how to locate peer-reviewed references and studies on sarcoidosis. We will begin by discussing research that has been summarized and is free to view by the public via the Internet. We then show you how to generate a bibliography on sarcoidosis and teach you how to keep current on new studies as they are published or undertaken by the scientific community.

The Combined Health Information Database

The Combined Health Information Database summarizes studies across numerous federal agencies. To limit your investigation to research studies and sarcoidosis, you will need to use the advanced search options. First, go to **http://chid.nih.gov/index.html**. From there, select the "Detailed Search" option (or go directly to that page with the following hyperlink: **http://chid.nih.gov/detail/detail.html**). The trick in extracting studies is found in the drop boxes at the bottom of the search page where "You may refine your search by." Select the dates and language you prefer, and the format option "Journal Article." At the top of the search form, select the number of records you would like to see (we recommend 100) and check the box to display "whole records." We recommend that you type in "sarcoidosis" (or synonyms) into the "For these words:" box. Consider using the option "anywhere in record" to make your search as broad as possible. If you want to limit the search to only a particular field, such as the title of the journal, then select this option in the "Search in these fields" drop box. The following is a sample of what you can expect from this type of search:

- **Practice Guidelines: American Thoracic Society Issues Consensus Statement on Sarcoidosis**

  Source: American Family Physician. 61(2): 553-554,556. January 15, 2000.

  Contact: American Academy of Family Physicians. 11400 Tomahawk Creek Parkway, Leawood, KS 66211-2672. (800) 274-2237 or (913) 906-6000. E-mail: fp@aafp.org. Website: www.aafp.org.

  Summary: This journal article provides health professionals with information on the consensus statement on sarcoidosis issued by the American Thoracic Society. This statement includes information on the epidemiology, pathogenesis, diagnosis, and treatment of sarcoidosis. According to the statement, sarcoidosis occurs mainly in adults younger than 40. The peak incidence occurs in the third decade of life. The clinical presentation and severity of the disease differ among ethnic and racial groups. Although various studies have examined the role of environmental or occupational factors in sarcoidosis, these factors require further investigation. Several lines of evidence suggest that sarcoidosis results from exposure of genetically susceptible persons to specific environmental agents. Nonspecific symptoms include fever, fatigue, malaise, and weight loss. Sarcoidosis may affect the pulmonary, lymphatic, hepatic, cutaneous, ocular, nervous, skeletal, and hematologic systems. Diagnosis involves a physical examination and laboratory tests. Treatment options include topical steroid therapy for mild manifestations and oral corticosteroids for systemic symptomatic disease. Other therapies include cytotoxic, antimalarial, and nonsteroidal anti-inflammatory agents.

- **Sarcoidosis and Systemic Vasculitis**

  Source: Seminars in Arthritis and Rheumatism. 30(1): 33-46. August 2000.

  Summary: This journal article provides health professionals with information on a retrospective study that reported on six cases of sarcoidosis and systemic vasculitis and compared clinicians' experiences with these six patients with experiences presented in the literature in English since 1966. The six patients had systemic illnesses that included fever, peripheral adenopathy, hilar adenopathy, rash, pulmonary parenchymal disease, musculoskeletal symptoms, and scleritis or iridocyclitis. Biopsies revealed features compatible with the diagnosis of sarcoidosis or necrotizing sarcoid granulomata in either skin, lymph node, lung, synovium, bone, bone marrow, liver, trachea, or sclera. Arteriography showed features of large vessel vasculitis in three patients, all of whom were African American, whereas patients with small vessel vasculitis were white. Prior reports of sarcoidosis-related vasculitis included 14 adults, half of whom had predominantly small vessel disease and half of whom had medium or large vessel disease. Eight previously reported children included seven with primarily large vessel sarcoid vasculitis. Racial background was noted in 15 reported cases and included 6 whites, 5 African Americans, and 4 Asians. Among the 6 patients in the retrospective study, 4 improved when treated with prednisone alone. However, relapses occurred when the drug was tapered or withdrawn. The article concludes that sarcoidosis may be complicated by systemic vasculitis that can affect small to large vessels. Sarcoid vasculitis can mimic hypersensitivity vasculitis, polyarteritis nodosa, microscopic polyangiitis, or Takayasu's arteritis. African American and Asian patients are disproportionately represented among cases with large vessel involvement. Corticosteroid and cytotoxic therapy is palliative for all forms of sarcoid vasculitis. However, relapses and morbidity from disease and treatment are common. 3 figures, 4 tables, and 42 references. (AA-M).

- **Sarcoidosis: A Primary Care Review**

Source: American Family Physician. 58(9): 2041-2050. December 1998.

Contact: American Academy of Family Physicians. 11400 Tomahawk Creek Parkway, Leawood, KS 66211-2672. (800) 274-2237 or (913) 906-6000. E-mail: fp@aafp.org. Website: www.aafp.org.

Summary: This journal article provides health professionals with information on the symptoms, diagnosis, and prognosis of sarcoidosis, as well as its treatment. This multisystemic disease of unknown etiology may affect any organ or system in the body and most commonly affects adults between 20 and 40 years of age. Patients with sarcoidosis frequently present with bilateral hilar lymphadenopathy and pulmonary infiltration, and they often have ocular and skin lesions. Skin manifestations can be either specific or nonspecific, but most are granulomatous and occur more commonly in African American patients. Ocular disease affects approximately one quarter of patients with systemic sarcoidosis and may involve any area of the eye. Other organs that may be affected are the kidneys, liver, heart, and central nervous system. Bone involvement may also occur. The diagnosis is established when clinical and radiographic findings are supported by histologic evidence of noncaseating epithelioid cell granulomas found on tissue biopsy. Diagnosis of sarcoidosis requires exclusion of other causes of granuloma formation. Sarcoidosis is also characterized by distinctive laboratory abnormalities, including hyperglobulinemia, an elevated serum angiotensin converting enzyme level, evidence of depressed cellular immunity manifested by cutaneous anergy, and, occasionally, hypercalcemia and hypercalciuria. Although glucocorticoids are the mainstay of therapy when treatment is required, other anti-inflammatory agents are being increasingly used. The prognosis is generally good, with spontaneous resolution of the disease as the rule. The article includes a case study. 8 figures, 1 table, and 10 references. (AA-M).

- **You Have Sarcoidosis: What Does This Mean to You?**

Source: American Family Physician. 58(9): 2051-2052. December 1998.

Contact: American Academy of Family Physicians. 11400 Tomahawk Creek Parkway, Leawood, KS 66211-2672. (800) 274-2237 or (913) 906-6000. E-mail: fp@aafp.org. Website: www.aafp.org.

Summary: This journal article uses a question and answer format to provide people who have sarcoidosis with information on this disease that may affect any organ or system in the body. Its cause is unknown. The disease, which most commonly affects adults aged 20 to 40 years old, is found more often in women than in men. The symptoms vary, depending on the part of the body affected. In most cases, the lungs are affected, but skin lesions occur in about one third to one half of those with sarcoidosis. Other common sites include the eye, kidney, and heart. Less common sites are the liver and bones. Diagnosis is based on a physical examination and various diagnostic tests. Treatment options include using corticosteroids or other medications. In many people, the disease improves without treatment.

- **Sarcoidosis of the Liver**

Source: Liver Update. 5(1): 6. Spring 1991.

Contact: Available from American Liver Foundation. 1425 Pompton Avenue, Cedar Grove, NJ 07009. (201) 256-2550 or (800) 223-0179.

Summary: Sarcoidosis is a multisystem disease of unknown etiology, characterized b y noncaseating granulomas that involve two or more organs. This brief article discusses sarcoidosis of the liver and reports on a study of 100 liver biopsies from 100 patients diagnosed with sarcoidosis. The author stresses that sarcoidosis may represent an important cause of cholestatic liver disease that is underreported.

- **Protean Face of Renal Sarcoidosis**

Source: JASN. Journal of the American Society of Nephrology. 12(3): 616-623. March 2001.

Contact: Available from Lippincott Williams and Wilkins. 12107 Insurance Way, Hagerstown, MD 21740. (800) 638-6423.

Summary: This article reviews renal (kidney) sarcoidosis, one manifestation of this multisystem granulomatous disorder of unknown cause. The disease is characterized by the presence of noncaseating epithelioid granulomas in involved organs. The cause of sarcoidosis remains to be determined; an infectious cause has been postulated since the disease was first described but has not been secured convincingly. Clinically important renal involvement is only an occasional problem in sarcoidosis. However, sarcoidosis can be a factor in renal stone disease (abnormal calcium homeostasis, or balance). The chronic hypercalcemia (too much calcium in the blood) and hypercalciuria (too much calcium in the urine) that can accompany sarcoidosis can lead to kidney insufficiency. Also, approximately 20 percent of patients with sarcoidosis show granulomatous inflammation in the kidney. Glomerular (the bundles of filtering nephrons in the kidney) involvement in sarcoidosis is not common, although various problems including membranous glomerulonephritis, IgA nephropathy, and focal segmental sclerosis have all been described. For each of these manifestations, the authors present a brief case report that illustrates the patient presentation and management issues. A final section notes that transplantation is not precluded in patients with sarcoidosis, although the condition may recur. Because lymph nodes throughout the body may enlarge, ureteral obstruction and retroperitoneal fibrosis have been described. The authors conclude that sarcoidosis offers a challenge to the nephrologist. 6 figures. 61 references.

- **Parotid Sarcoidosis Mimicking Sjogren's Syndrome: Report of a Case**

Source: Journal of Oral and Maxillofacial Surgery. 60(1): 117-120. January 2002.

Contact: Available from W.B. Saunders Company. Periodicals Department, P.O. Box 629239, Orlando, FL 32862-8239. (800) 654-2452. Website: www.harcourthealth.com.

Summary: Sarcoidosis is a disease that commonly occurs in young or middle aged adults and frequently affects the hilar lymph nodes, lungs, eyes, and skin. Because parotid gland (salivary gland) enlargement is a common clinical problem, the diagnosis of sarcoidosis can be difficult. This article describes a case of chronic sarcoidosis showing clinical symptoms that could represent both Sjogren's syndrome and Lofgren's syndrome. Besides the diffuse enlargement of the parotid glands affected by sarcoidosis (seen with ultrasound), there are granulomatous changes in the glandular parenchyma (the body of the gland itself) that cannot be detected clinically. These findings allow the distinction of sarcoidosis from several other causes for chronic, painless parotid enlargement, especially Sjogren's syndrome, which typically presents with a specific pattern of multiple, scattered cystic changes in the parenchyma. The need for treatment depends on the stage of the disease and the kind of organic changes. 4 figures. 22 references.

- **Oral Manifestations of Sarcoidosis**

  Source: Oral Surgery, Oral Medicine, Oral Pathology, Oral Radiology, and Endodontics. 83(4): 458-461. April 1997.

  Summary: The authors report two new cases of sarcoidosis of the buccal mucosa and analyze the literature on the oral manifestations of sarcoidosis. The analysis of 45 cases of oral sarcoidosis (43 from the literature and the 2 new presented cases) revealed 12 lesions in the jaws, 10 in the buccal mucosa, 6 in the gingiva, 5 in the lips, 5 in the floor of the mouth, 4 in the tongue, and 3 in the palate. Sarcoidosis in the jaw was located in the alveolar bone and presented as an ill-defined radiolucency. Submucosal nodules were observed in sarcoidosis affecting the buccal mucosa, palate, and lip. Swelling was the main manifestation in the gingiva. In the floor of the mouth, sarcoidosis presented as ranula and that of the tongue as induration. In most of the cases, the lesions in the buccal mucosa, gingiva, and tongue were the first clinical manifestation of the disease. The authors conclude that oral sarcoidosis lesions should be considered in the differential diagnosis of oral soft tissue swellings and jaw lesions. 3 figures. 53 references. (AA-M).

Federally-Funded Research on Sarcoidosis

The U.S. Government supports a variety of research studies relating to sarcoidosis and associated conditions. These studies are tracked by the Office of Extramural Research at the National Institutes of Health.[19] CRISP (Computerized Retrieval of Information on Scientific Projects) is a searchable database of federally-funded biomedical research projects conducted at universities, hospitals, and other institutions. Visit the CRISP Web site at **http://commons.cit.nih.gov/crisp3/CRISP.Generate_Ticket**. You can perform targeted searches by various criteria including geography, date, as well as topics related to sarcoidosis and related conditions.

For most of the studies, the agencies reporting into CRISP provide summaries or abstracts. As opposed to clinical trial research using patients, many federally-funded studies use animals or simulated models to explore sarcoidosis and related conditions. In some cases, therefore, it may be difficult to understand how some basic or fundamental research could eventually translate into medical practice. The following sample is typical of the type of information found when searching the CRISP database for sarcoidosis:

- **Project Title: Case Control Etiologic Study of Sarcoidosis**

  Principal Investigator & Institution: Rossman, Milton; ; University of Pennsylvania 1 College Hall Philadelphia, Pa 19104

  Timing: Fiscal Year 2000

  Summary: Ten clinical centers in the United States are recruiting cases for an NIH sponsored study titled "A Case Control Etiologic Study of Sarcoidosis." The objectives include: 1) to test hypotheses concerning environmental, occupational, lifestyle, and other risk factors for sarcoidosis, 2) examine the familial aggregation of sarcoidosis, 3) To test genetic hypotheses concerning aggregation of sarcoidosis, 4) To describe the natural history of sarcoidosis, particularly among groups such as African-Americans who appear to be disproportionately affected, 5) To identify risk factors for progression to more sever disease and 6(To implement a system for storing biological specimens including blood cells, plasma, and serum from cases and control subjects and bronchoalveolar lavage fluid and cells from a well characterized series of cases of sarcoidosis which represent the spectrum from mild to severe disease.

  Website: http://commons.cit.nih.gov/crisp3/CRISP.Generate_Ticket

---

[19] Healthcare projects are funded by the National Institutes of Health (NIH), Substance Abuse and Mental Health Services (SAMHSA), Health Resources and Services Administration (HRSA), Food and Drug Administration (FDA), Centers for Disease Control and Prevention (CDCP), Agency for Healthcare Research and Quality (AHRQ), and Office of Assistant Secretary of Health (OASH).

- **Project Title: Case Control Etiologic Study of Sarcoidosis**

  Principal Investigator & Institution: Newman, Lee; ; University of Colorado Hlth Sciences Ctr 4200 E 9Th Ave Denver, Co 80262

  Timing: Fiscal Year 2000

  Summary: Sarcoidosis is a chronic disease that often involves the lungs; its cause is unknown. The ACCESS Study (A Case Control Etiologic Study of Sarcoidosis) will compare facts about patients with sarcoidosis (cases) and people without sarcoidosis (controls) to learn what causes the disease. Ten clinic research centers from across America are in this study. The ACCESS Study is a research project of the National Institutes of Health. The ten clinics will enroll a total of 720 cases for the study. Also, 720 controls will enroll in the study. Data and blood samples will be collected from the controls to compare with the data and blood samples from patients with sarcoidosis. Only patients with newly found sarcoidosis, on biopsy, are asked to join this study. If these patients agree to participate, there will be five parts of this study. First is an interview to record medical, environmental, and family history. Second is a physical examination by a doctor on the research team. Third, clinic staff will take a sample of the patient's blood. Fourth, clinic staff will perform or review the results of tests that are part of the usual care for sarcoidosis. Fifth, clinic staff will contact cases every six months for two years and see them in the clinic two years after they join the study. This follow-up appointment two years after the initial visit will require one to two hours of time. Cases and controls will be paid for their time and effort participating in ACCESS. None of the testing costs will be passed onto a case or control. Potential causes of sarcoidosis which are explored in this study are genetic predispositions, occupational and environmental exposures, place of residence, medication usage, and organ involvement and what it means for disease stability or progression. The cause of sarcoidosis may not prove to be a single, known exposure. Interactions of exposures with genetic predispositions would have important implications for our understanding of immune system responses as well as the origin and development of sarcoidosis.

  Website: http://commons.cit.nih.gov/crisp3/CRISP.Generate_Ticket

- **Project Title: Clinical Center for Etiology of Sarcoidosis--A Case Control Study**

  Principal Investigator & Institution: Judson, Marc A.; ; Medical University of South Carolina 171 Ashley Ave Charleston, Sc 29403

  Timing: Fiscal Year 2000

Summary: The case control study is designed to investigate possible cause and risk factors for sarcoidosis. Evaluation of cases and controls to determine the etiology of sarcoidosis will include an inquiry into environmental and occupational exposures, family history, medical history, and collection of blood specimens. Blood specimens will be used to identify potential immunogenetic and infectious contributions to sarcoidosis by means of specialized studies involving recently developed microbiology and nucleic acid analysis techniques such as HLA Class II marker studies, mycobacterial studies, immunogenetic studies, differential display polymerase chain reactin (PCR) studies, and comparisons of nucleic acid sequences from blood specimens to those of known pathogens. Bronchoalveolar lavage studies will also be performed. Specific hypothesis to be addressed include that genetic factors, infections, and occupational or environmental factors affect risk for sarcoidosis. The clinical course study of 240 cases is designed to: (1) define sarcoidosis cases that do or do not clinically resolve over a two-year period of follow-up, and (2) develop a clinical / radiographical / physiologic sarcoidosis assessment system for reporting the severity of disease.

Website: http://commons.cit.nih.gov/crisp3/CRISP.Generate_Ticket

- **Project Title: Core--Data Coordination**

Principal Investigator & Institution: Fowler, Sarah E.; ; Case Western Reserve Univ-Henry Ford Hsc Henry Ford Health Science Ctr Detroit, Mi 48202

Timing: Fiscal Year 2000

Summary: Sarcoidosis is a systemic granulomatous disease of unknown etiology that likely involves exposure to some environmental agent in a genetically susceptible host. We propose to identify sarcoidosis susceptibility genes and determine how these genes and environmental risk factors interact to cause sarcoidosis. This will be accomplished by organizing a multicenter consortium to recruit an adequate sample of sarcoidosis families for analysis. We plan to use affecting sibling pair linkage analysis to scan the genome for linked chromosomal regions, transmission disequilibrium testing to evaluate candidate genes in those regions with evidence for linkage and an environmental questionnaire to collect data to test for possible interactions of susceptibility genes with exogenous risk factors. This application offers the Department of Biostatistics and Research Epidemiology, Henry Ford Health System as the Data Coordinating Center (DCC) for the project. The DCC will provide administrative coordination, develop study documents, develop recruitment strategies, provide study tracking, establish a central data base, conduct data quality assurance, and collaborate with other members of the consortium in analysis of the results of the study. The Data Coordinating Center (DCC) will be an independent unit within the consortium, and will take guidance from the Steering Committee. The DCC team is headed by Principal Investigator Sarah Fowler, PhD, a senior biostatistical who specializes in coordinating centers for multi-center studies, and coordinating center biostatistician and Co-PI Mei Lu, PhD, who will sere as project manger for the DCC. DCC Co-Investigator Marvella Ford, PhD, will advise the collaborative group on the recruitment and retention of African American subjects and their families. The Coordinating Center team also includes a support staff consisting of individuals (programmer, data coordinator and secretary) experienced in and dedicated to methodologies for multi-center studies.

Website: http://commons.cit.nih.gov/crisp3/CRISP.Generate_Ticket

- **Project Title: Etiology of Sarcoidosis a Case Control Study**

Principal Investigator & Institution: Teirstein, Alvin; Medicine; Mount Sinai School of Medicine of Nyu of New York University New York, Ny 10029

Timing: Fiscal Year 2000; Project Start 7-JUL-1995; Project End 6-MAY-2001

Summary: The overall objective of this program is to support a multicenter case- control study on the potential etiologic factors for sarcoidosis. Cases will also be followed to gain information on the natural history of this disease including risk factors for progression of disease. A steering committee will develop a protocol and manual of operations which will address the most promising hypotheses to be pursued to identify the cause(s) of sarcoidosis. The protocol will include a comprehensive clinical characterization of each participant and determination of markers of immune responsiveness. The contractor will participate in a system for banking biological specimens. A clinical coordinating center will be established to collect, manage and analyze the data from the clinical centers. It is estimated that the total study population will consist of 720 cases and 1,440 controls. It is estimated that each clinical center will enroll, interview, and examine 72 cases (age 21 years or older) with sarcoidosis and, enroll, interview and collect a blood specimen from 144 matched control subjects over a four year period. Clinical centers will 1) test specific hypotheses involving risk factors, familial aggregation, and genetics of the etiology of this disease and 2) describe the natural history of sarcoidosis. A six year schedule is envisioned as follows: Phase I (12 Months): A collaborative protocol and manual of operations will be developed; Phase II (48 Months): will involve the recruitment and follow-up of patients and recruitment and interviewing of control subjects, and Phase III (12 Months): will involve data analysis.

Website: http://commons.cit.nih.gov/crisp3/CRISP.Generate_Ticket

- **Project Title: Genetic Epidemiology of Sarcoidosis**

Principal Investigator & Institution: Iannuzzi, Michael C.; Professor; Medicine; Case Western Reserve Univ-Henry Ford Hsc Henry Ford Health Science Ctr Detroit, Mi 48202

Timing: Fiscal Year 2000; Project Start 1-DEC-1996; Project End 0-NOV-2000

Summary: (Adapted from Investigator's Abstract) Sarcoidosis is a multisystem, granulomatous inflammatory disease of unknown etiology. Hereditary susceptibility to sarcoidosis is suggested by reports of familial clustering and a higher prevalence in certain ethnic groups, particularly African Americans. Over four hundred kindreds been reported in the medical literature and these investigators have recently described 101 families and shown that African Americans have a higher prevalence rate of familial sarcoidosis than Caucasians (19% vs. 5%). The reasons why sarcoidosis clusters in families or the role of genetic factors in this disease are not known. The objectives of this proposal are to determine if hereditary susceptibility predisposes African Americans to sarcoidosis and to identify sarcoidosis susceptibility genes in African Americans. The study will be carried out in African American families ascertained through 400 African American sarcoidosis patients evaluated at the Henry Ford Health System. They plan to test for association of sarcoidosis with markers for candidate genes using the affected family-based control method and test for possible environmental risk factors and genetic mechanisms of disease transmission by performing a segregation analysis in African American families. If one or more of the candidate genes studied show a strong association with sarcoidosis or if there is an indication of major gene segregation for the disease, they will be well positioned for future linkage studies. Investigating the hereditary susceptibility of sarcoidosis can best be done in African Americans, because of the greater severity and occurrence of disease in this population. Once the reasons for familial aggregation of sarcoidosis are determined, the investigators state that the etiology of this disease will be better understood and suitable prevention and treatment should be able to be designed.

Website: http://commons.cit.nih.gov/crisp3/CRISP.Generate_Ticket

- **Project Title: Genetics of Actinic Prurigo**

  Principal Investigator & Institution: Elston, Robert C.; Professor; Case Western Reserve University 10900 Euclid Ave Cleveland, Oh 44106

  Timing: Fiscal Year 2000

  Summary: Sarcoidosis is a multisystem granulomatous inflammatory disease of unknown etiology. Hereditary susceptibility to sarcoidosis is suggested by reports of familial clustering and a higher prevalence in certain ethnic groups, particularly African-Americans. Candidate genes for the granulomatous inflammatory disorders, Blau syndrome and Crohn's disease have been localized to the centrometric region of chromosome 16. We therefore investigated whether this region is also involved in sarcoidosis. Using a sample of 35 African-American affected sibling pairs, we found no evidence of linkage in this general region, and could exclude from it a dominant gene with relative risk < 5, or a recessive gene with relative risk < 3, causing sarcoidosis. In particular, we concluded that the Blau syndrome gene does not have a major effect on sarcoidosis susceptibility. We plan to test for association of sarcoidosis with markers for other candidate genes and to perform a segregation analysis in order to test simultaneously for possible environmental risk factors and genetic mechanisms of disease transmission. This study is ongoing.

  Website: http://commons.cit.nih.gov/crisp3/CRISP.Generate_Ticket

- **Project Title: Pilot Investigation of Safety and Efficacy of Thalidomide in Sarcoidosis**

  Principal Investigator & Institution: Oliver, Stephen J.; ; Rockefeller University 66Th and York Ave New York, Ny 10021

  Timing: Fiscal Year 2000

  Summary: Sarcoidosis is a multisystem disease of unknown etiology characterized by the formation of noncaseating granulomas. Disease involvement can be self limited or chronic, ranging from asymptomatic to end organ failure. The disease may affect lungs, thoracic lymph nodes, skin, eyes, and other organs. Corticosteroids remain the primary sarcoidosis therapy. However, steroid treatment has multiple side effects and may fail to alter the disease course. The proinflammatory cytokine TNF-alpha may play an important role in mediating sarcoid disease activity. TNF-alpha production by activated macrophages is an important element in the cell mediated immune response leading to granuloma formation. Serum levels of TNF-alpha and soluble TNF-alpha receptors are elevated in sarcoidosis patients and correlate with disease activity. Thalidomide, an inhibitor of TNF-alpha production, has been shown to have both anti-inflammatory and immune modulating effects in a number of autoimmune diseases, including discoid lupus, aphthous ulcer formation, erythema nodosum leprosum, and others. The addition of thalidomide to antibiotic regimens has also improved morbidity and mortality in animal models of M. tuberculosis infection of the pulmonary and central nervous systems. This study will evaluate the effect of daily thalidomide administration in sarcoidosis patients over a 4 month period, using clinical and laboratory based disease activity measures. Serially recorded clinical disease activity measures include spirometry, skin photographs, erythrocyte sedimentation rates, Health Assessment Questionnaires, and joint counts. Chest x-rays and several skin biopsies will be performed at several defined time points. Laboratory based disease activity measures include plasma TNF-alpha and soluble TNF-alpha receptor, soluble interleukin 2 receptor, and intercellular cell adhesion molecule-1. Interferon gamma plasma levels will also be determined. T-lymphocytes subsets and antigen-stimulated lymphocyte proliferation will be measured. Drug safety in this patient group will be monitored by blood chemistries and cell counts, history and physical exams, and renal function assessments performed during monthly patient visits.

Website: http://commons.cit.nih.gov/crisp3/CRISP.Generate_Ticket

- **Project Title: Regulation of THL Responses in Pulmonary Sarcoidosis**

Principal Investigator & Institution: Moller, David R.; Associate Professor of Medicine; Medicine; Johns Hopkins University 3400 N Charles St Baltimore, Md 21218

Timing: Fiscal Year 2000; Project Start 1-MAY-1996; Project End 0-APR-2001

Summary: Sarcoidosis is a multisystem granulomatous disorder of unknown etiology that involves the lungs in over 90% of affected individuals. Chronic progressive pulmonary sarcoidosis can result in end-stage fibrosis and cor pulmonale. Treatment with corticosteroids may be toxic and ineffective. As many as 5% of individuals with pulmonary sarcoidosis die of causes directly related to the disease. With an incidence in the U.S. of 11-4- per 100,000 people, sarcoidosis represents a significant health problem. The overall objective of this proposal is to further our understanding of the immunologic and inflammatory processes mediating granulomatous inflammation in pulmonary sarcoidosis. T-cells are involved in the pathogenesis of the disease since "activated", lymphokine-releasing CD4+ T- cells accumulate at sites of disease such as the lung. The accumulation of these T-cells in the lung is selective and oligoclonal, characterized by the preferential usage of T-cell response. Analysis of the pattern of cytokines expressed in the sarcoid lung have demonstrated that IFNgamma and to a lesser extent, IL2 are strongly expressed while IL4 and IL5 are expressed at very low or nondetectable levels. This polarization towards a Th1 immune response is likely playing a key role in the development and perpetuation of granulomatous inflammation in sarcoidosis since Th1 responses are critical in mediating cell-mediated immune responses in many infectious and autoimmune diseases. Our preliminary data demonstrate that IL12, a cytokine critical to the initiation of Th1 immune responses, is markedly upregulated in the sarcoid lung. The experiments proposed in this application are aimed at testing the hypothesis that sarcoidosis is a Th1-mediated disease driven by the dysregulated production of Il12. This hypothesis will be tested by studies with the following Specific Aims; 1) Determine whether polarization towards Th1 associated cytokine expression in characteristic of tissues affected by granulomatous inflammation in sarcoidosis, 2) characterize and compare the regulation of IL12 expression in sarcoid and normal human alveolar macrophages and peripheral blood, and 3) determine the role of IL12 in the Th1 deviation of immune responses in pulmonary sarcoidosis. These studies should increase our understanding of the processes controlling Th1 polarization in sarcoidosis and provide insights into the effects and regulatory determinants of chronic expression of Il12 in the human lung. Thus, these studies may assist in the development of new therapies designed to halt the granulomatous and fibrotic responses that lead to end-stage pulmonary disease in sarcoidosis.

Website: http://commons.cit.nih.gov/crisp3/CRISP.Generate_Ticket

- **Project Title: Sarcoidosis Genes**

    Principal Investigator & Institution: Reynolds, Herbert Y.; J. Lloyd Huck Professor of Medicine; Pennsylvania State Univ Hershey Med Ctr 500 University Dr Hershey, Pa 17033

    Timing: Fiscal Year 2000; Project Start 5-AUG-1995; Project End 0-NOV-2004

    Summary: The investigators wish to determine if any special genes can be identified in persons with sarcoidosis. Sarcoidosis is a multi-organ illness, involving the respiratory tract and less often other organs such as the liver, skin and eyes, that has no known cause but does seem to be present in families. A hereditary susceptibility to sarcoidosis seems possible.

    Website: http://commons.cit.nih.gov/crisp3/CRISP.Generate_Ticket

- **Project Title: T Lymphocyte Transendothelial Migration in Sarcoidosis**

Principal Investigator & Institution: Berman, Jeffrey S.; ; Boston University 121 Bay State Rd Boston, Ma 02215

Timing: Fiscal Year 2000

Summary: Lung sarcoidosis is characterized by a CD4+ (helper) T-lymphocyte lymphocytic alveolitis. The effector T-cells present in the lung in sarcoidosis produce cytokines, including interleukin (IL)-2 and interferon-gamma, which promote inflammation and maintain granuloma formation. The relative contributions to this CD4+ T-cell alveolitis of recruitment from the blood versus in situ proliferation in the lung are not clear. T-cell recruitment to tissue occurs by adherence of migration- prone to locally activated endothelial cells, interaction with matrix proteins and migration in response to locally produced chemoattractants. We have recently documented the presence of a specialized population of memory CD4+ and CD8+ T cells in normal human blood which are highly likely to migrate through normal or activated endothelial cells in an in vitro assay. These cells resemble cells which home to normal lung in terms of T- cell memory and activation markers. We have documented a marked increase in these migrating cells in the blood of a subset of patients with sarcoidosis and CD4-lymphocytic alveolitis. We hypothesize that these migrating cells are T-helper effector cells which modify granulomatous inflammation in sarcoidosis. We have also documented the presence of a novel CD4+ cell chemoattractant (lymphocyte chemoattractant factor, LCF/IL-16) in the bronchoalveolar lavage (BAL) of 4 patients with sarcoidosis. This chemoattractant was identified and cloned in our laboratory and is not found n the BAL of normal non-smokers. We hypothesize that CD4+ T cell recruitment from the blood plays a important role in pulmonary sarcoidosis, and that two interrelated processes contribute to increased CD4+ effector T cell recruitment to sites of granuloma formation: 1. Increased numbers of migration-prone effector T- cells into the blood where they are available to home to lung or other inflammatory sites, and once in tissue contribute to inflammation, resolution and fibrosis, and 2. Production of CD4+ T cell specify chemoattractants, including LCF. We are presently testing this hypothesis by: 1. Documenting the presence, phenotype and function (cytokine production) of migrating T cells from peripheral blood of normals versa patients with sarcoidosis; and 2. Surveying tissues, lung cells and lavage samples from patients with sarcoidosis or the presence of LCF/IL-16. We will also examine the effect of several known or proposed therapies for sarcoidosis on the adhesion and transendothelial migration of CD4+ T cells from the blood of normals and patients with sarcoidosis. These studies may provide insight into the mechanisms by which granulomas are maintained in sarcoidosis, and may suggest new forms of specific therapy targeted at effector cell recruitment.

Website: http://commons.cit.nih.gov/crisp3/CRISP.Generate_Ticket

E-Journals: PubMed Central[20]

PubMed Central (PMC) is a digital archive of life sciences journal literature developed and managed by the National Center for Biotechnology Information (NCBI) at the U.S. National Library of Medicine (NLM).[21] Access to this growing archive of e-journals is free and unrestricted.[22] To search, go to **http://www.pubmedcentral.nih.gov/index.html#search**, and type "sarcoidosis" (or synonyms) into the search box. This search gives you access to full-text articles. The following is a sample of items found for sarcoidosis in the PubMed Central database:

- **Cardiac Involvement in Sarcoidosis** by Panayotis Fasseas, Kathleen M. Galatro, Biana Leybishkis, and Billie Fyfe; 2001
  http://www.pubmedcentral.nih.gov/articlerender.fcgi?artid=101160

- **Genotyping in the MHC locus: potential for defining predictive markers in sarcoidosis** by Ulrike Seitzer, Johannes Gerdes, and Joachim Muller-Quernheim; 2002
  http://www.pubmedcentral.nih.gov/articlerender.fcgi?artid=64817

- **T-Cell Receptor Variable Region Gene Usage by CD4+ and CD8+ T Cells in Bronchoalveolar Lavage Fluid and Peripheral Blood of Sarcoidosis Patients** by J Grunewald, O Olerup, U Persson, MB Ohrn, H Wigzell, and A Eklund; 1994 May 24
  http://www.pubmedcentral.nih.gov/articlerender.fcgi?rendertype=abstract&artid=43910

---

[20] Adapted from the National Library of Medicine:
http://www.pubmedcentral.nih.gov/about/intro.html.

[21] With PubMed Central, NCBI is taking the lead in preservation and maintenance of open access to electronic literature, just as NLM has done for decades with printed biomedical literature. PubMed Central aims to become a world-class library of the digital age.

[22] The value of PubMed Central, in addition to its role as an archive, lies the availability of data from diverse sources stored in a common format in a single repository. Many journals already have online publishing operations, and there is a growing tendency to publish material online only, to the exclusion of print.

The National Library of Medicine: PubMed

One of the quickest and most comprehensive ways to find academic studies in both English and other languages is to use PubMed, maintained by the National Library of Medicine. The advantage of PubMed over previously mentioned sources is that it covers a greater number of domestic and foreign references. It is also free to the public.[23] If the publisher has a Web site that offers full text of its journals, PubMed will provide links to that site, as well as to sites offering other related data. User registration, a subscription fee, or some other type of fee may be required to access the full text of articles in some journals.

To generate your own bibliography of studies dealing with sarcoidosis, simply go to the PubMed Web site at **www.ncbi.nlm.nih.gov/pubmed**. Type "sarcoidosis" (or synonyms) into the search box, and click "Go." The following is the type of output you can expect from PubMed for "sarcoidosis" (hyperlinks lead to article summaries):

- **Spontaneous remission or response to methotrexate in sarcoidosis.**
  Author(s): Lacher MJ.
  Source: Annals of Internal Medicine. 1968 December; 69(6): 1247-8. No Abstract Available.
  http://www.ncbi.nlm.nih.gov:80/entrez/query.fcgi?cmd=Retrieve&db=PubMed&list_uids=5725738&dopt=Abstract

Vocabulary Builder

Antibiotic: A drug that kills or inhibits the growth of bacteria. [NIH]

Arteriography: Roentgenography of arteries after injection of radiopacque material into the blood stream. [EU]

Assay: Determination of the amount of a particular constituent of a mixture, or of the biological or pharmacological potency of a drug. [EU]

Asymptomatic: Showing or causing no symptoms. [EU]

Bilateral: Having two sides, or pertaining to both sides. [EU]

Buccal: Pertaining to or directed toward the cheek. In dental anatomy, used

---

[23] PubMed was developed by the National Center for Biotechnology Information (NCBI) at the National Library of Medicine (NLM) at the National Institutes of Health (NIH). The PubMed database was developed in conjunction with publishers of biomedical literature as a search tool for accessing literature citations and linking to full-text journal articles at Web sites of participating publishers. Publishers that participate in PubMed supply NLM with their citations electronically prior to or at the time of publication.

to refer to the buccal surface of a tooth. [EU]

Carcinoma: A malignant new growth made up of epithelial cells tending to infiltrate the surrounding tissues and give rise to metastases. [EU]

Chromosomal: Pertaining to chromosomes. [EU]

Cutaneous: Pertaining to the skin; dermal; dermic. [EU]

Cytotoxic: Pertaining to or exhibiting cytotoxicity. [EU]

Dermatology: A medical specialty concerned with the skin, its structure, functions, diseases, and treatment. [NIH]

Discoid: Shaped like a disk. [EU]

Efficacy: The extent to which a specific intervention, procedure, regimen, or service produces a beneficial result under ideal conditions. Ideally, the determination of efficacy is based on the results of a randomized control trial. [NIH]

Erythrocytes: Red blood cells. Mature erythrocytes are non-nucleated, biconcave disks containing hemoglobin whose function is to transport oxygen. [NIH]

Glomerular: Pertaining to or of the nature of a glomerulus, especially a renal glomerulus. [EU]

Glomerulonephritis: A variety of nephritis characterized by inflammation of the capillary loops in the glomeruli of the kidney. It occurs in acute, subacute, and chronic forms and may be secondary to haemolytic streptococcal infection. Evidence also supports possible immune or autoimmune mechanisms. [EU]

Hematology: A subspecialty of internal medicine concerned with morphology, physiology, and pathology of the blood and blood-forming tissues. [NIH]

Hepatic: Pertaining to the liver. [EU]

Homeostasis: A tendency to stability in the normal body states (internal environment) of the organism. It is achieved by a system of control mechanisms activated by negative feedback; e.g. a high level of carbon dioxide in extracellular fluid triggers increased pulmonary ventilation, which in turn causes a decrease in carbon dioxide concentration. [EU]

Hypercalcemia: Abnormally high level of calcium in the blood. [NIH]

Induration: 1. the quality of being hard; the process of hardening. 2. an abnormally hard spot or place. [EU]

Infiltration: The diffusion or accumulation in a tissue or cells of substances not normal to it or in amounts of the normal. Also, the material so accumulated. [EU]

Intestinal: Pertaining to the intestine. [EU]

Iridocyclitis: Inflammation of the iris and of the ciliary body; anterior uveitis. [EU]

Lesion: Any pathological or traumatic discontinuity of tissue or loss of function of a part. [EU]

LH: A small glycoprotein hormone secreted by the anterior pituitary. LH plays an important role in controlling ovulation and in controlling secretion of hormones by the ovaries and testes. [NIH]

Lupus: A form of cutaneous tuberculosis. It is seen predominantly in women and typically involves the nasal, buccal, and conjunctival mucosa. [NIH]

Lymphadenopathy: Disease of the lymph nodes. [EU]

Lymphocytic: Pertaining to, characterized by, or of the nature of lymphocytes. [EU]

Malaise: A vague feeling of bodily discomfort. [EU]

Microbiology: The study of microorganisms such as fungi, bacteria, algae, archaea, and viruses. [NIH]

Monocytes: Large, phagocytic mononuclear leukocytes produced in the vertebrate bone marrow and released into the blood; contain a large, oval or somewhat indented nucleus surrounded by voluminous cytoplasm and numerous organelles. [NIH]

Mucosa: A mucous membrane, or tunica mucosa. [EU]

Nephrology: A subspecialty of internal medicine concerned with the anatomy, physiology, and pathology of the kidney. [NIH]

Nephrons: The functional units of the kidney, consisting of the glomerulus and the attached tubule. [NIH]

Nephropathy: Disease of the kidneys. [EU]

Ocular: 1. of, pertaining to, or affecting the eye. 2. eyepiece. [EU]

Palliative: 1. affording relief, but not cure. 2. an alleviating medicine. [EU]

Pathogenesis: The cellular events and reactions that occur in the development of disease. [NIH]

Phenotype: The entire physical, biochemical, and physiological makeup of an individual as determined by his or her genes and by the environment in the broad sense. [NIH]

Physiologic: Normal; not pathologic; characteristic of or conforming to the normal functioning or state of the body or a tissue or organ; physiological. [EU]

Predisposition: A latent susceptibility to disease which may be activated under certain conditions, as by stress. [EU]

Receptor: 1. a molecular structure within a cell or on the surface characterized by (1) selective binding of a specific substance and (2) a specific physiologic effect that accompanies the binding, e.g., cell-surface receptors for peptide hormones, neurotransmitters, antigens, complement fragments, and immunoglobulins and cytoplasmic receptors for steroid hormones. 2. a sensory nerve terminal that responds to stimuli of various kinds. [EU]

Remission: A diminution or abatement of the symptoms of a disease; also the period during which such diminution occurs. [EU]

Sclerosis: A induration, or hardening; especially hardening of a part from inflammation and in diseases of the interstitial substance. The term is used chiefly for such a hardening of the nervous system due to hyperplasia of the connective tissue or to designate hardening of the blood vessels. [EU]

Sedimentation: The act of causing the deposit of sediment, especially by the use of a centrifugal machine. [EU]

Spirometry: Measurement of volume of air inhaled or exhaled by the lung. [NIH]

Symptomatic: 1. pertaining to or of the nature of a symptom. 2. indicative (of a particular disease or disorder). 3. exhibiting the symptoms of a particular disease but having a different cause. 4. directed at the allying of symptoms, as symptomatic treatment. [EU]

Testis: Either of the paired male reproductive glands that produce the male germ cells and the male hormones. [NIH]

Thalidomide: A pharmaceutical agent originally introduced as a non-barbiturate hypnotic, but withdrawn from the market because of its known tetratogenic effects. It has been reintroduced and used for a number of immunological and inflammatory disorders. Thalidomide displays immunosuppresive and anti-angiogenic activity. It inhibits release of tumor necrosis factor alpha from monocytes, and modulates other cytokine action. [NIH]

Thoracic: Pertaining to or affecting the chest. [EU]

Thrombocytopenia: Decrease in the number of blood platelets. [EU]

Topical: Pertaining to a particular surface area, as a topical anti-infective applied to a certain area of the skin and affecting only the area to which it is applied. [EU]

Trachea: The cartilaginous and membranous tube descending from the larynx and branching into the right and left main bronchi. [NIH]

Vasculitis: Inflammation of a vessel, angiitis. [EU]

CHAPTER 5. PATENTS ON SARCOIDOSIS

Overview

You can learn about innovations relating to sarcoidosis by reading recent patents and patent applications. Patents can be physical innovations (e.g. chemicals, pharmaceuticals, medical equipment) or processes (e.g. treatments or diagnostic procedures). The United States Patent and Trademark Office defines a patent as a grant of a property right to the inventor, issued by the Patent and Trademark Office.[24] Patents, therefore, are intellectual property. For the United States, the term of a new patent is 20 years from the date when the patent application was filed. If the inventor wishes to receive economic benefits, it is likely that the invention will become commercially available to patients with sarcoidosis within 20 years of the initial filing. It is important to understand, therefore, that an inventor's patent does not indicate that a product or service is or will be commercially available to patients with sarcoidosis. The patent implies only that the inventor has "the right to exclude others from making, using, offering for sale, or selling" the invention in the United States. While this relates to U.S. patents, similar rules govern foreign patents.

In this chapter, we show you how to locate information on patents and their inventors. If you find a patent that is particularly interesting to you, contact the inventor or the assignee for further information.

---

[24]Adapted from The U. S. Patent and Trademark Office:
http://www.uspto.gov/web/offices/pac/doc/general/whatis.htm.

Patents on Sarcoidosis

By performing a patent search focusing on sarcoidosis, you can obtain information such as the title of the invention, the names of the inventor(s), the assignee(s) or the company that owns or controls the patent, a short abstract that summarizes the patent, and a few excerpts from the description of the patent. The abstract of a patent tends to be more technical in nature, while the description is often written for the public. Full patent descriptions contain much more information than is presented here (e.g. claims, references, figures, diagrams, etc.). We will tell you how to obtain this information later in the chapter. The following is an example of the type of information that you can expect to obtain from a patent search on sarcoidosis:

- **Method employing imiquimod cream for treatment of topical sarcoidosis on equine**

  Inventor(s): Brenman; Steven A. (4960 S. Lafayette La., Cherry Hills, CO 80110)

  Assignee(s): none reported

  Patent Number: 6,147,086

  Date filed: September 1, 1999

  Abstract: A method for the treatment of topical sarcoidosis on equine includes providing a therapeutic substance substantially in the form of an imiquimod 5% cream and applying the therapeutic substance a plurality of times spaced at intervals from one another to an outer surface of the body of an equine such that the therapeutic substance substantially covers symptomatic manifestations of topical sarcoidosis on the outer surface of the equine body.

  Excerpt(s): The present invention generally relates to topical sarcoidosis and, more particularly, is concerned with a method employing an imiquimod cream for the treatment of topical sarcoidosis on equine. ... Sarcoidosis is an ailment of equine, such as horses, donkeys and mules. Sarcoidosis is most commonly topical in nature. Sarcoids are the typical symptomatic manifestations of sarcoidosis. Sarcoids are tumors which are nonmetastatic. Sarcoids are formed by proliferation of neoplastic fibroblasts which results in the thickening or ulceration of skin. Sarcoids may occur alone or in clusters. Sarcoids commonly arise on the head, limbs and abdomen, but can occur anywhere on the body of a horse. Sarcoids are the most frequently found tumor of horses. Though not life threatening, sarcoids generally reduce the value of a horse because their location on the horse adversely affects the performance of the horse when employed for various activities. Sarcoidosis is believed to be caused by infection of the bovine papilloma virus. ... A variety of treatments for topical sarcoidosis have been tried over the years, including surgical excision, cryotherapy, immunotherapy, radiotherapy, laser therapy, hyperthermia and topical and intratumoral chemotherapy. Surgical excision involves the use of surgical techniques to cut and remove sarcoids from adjacent healthy tissue. Cryotherapy involves freezing sarcoids. A refrigerant, commonly liquid nitrogen, is sprayed on the sarcoids to kill the cells of the tumors. Immunotherapy involves the use of antigens to stimulate lymphocytes and to increase natural killer cells of the host animal to kill the cells of the sarcoids. An attenuated strain of Mycobacterium bovis is commonly used in this procedure. Radiotherapy involves the use of radiation to kill the cells of the sarcoids. Radioactive isotopes are used to deliver a continuous and high dose of radiation locally to each tumor without affecting adjacent healthy tissue. Laser therapy involves cutting and evaporating sarcoids with a laser. Carbon dioxide lasers are commonly used for this procedure. Hyperthermia involves heating the tumor cells to kill them. The hyperthermia is commonly induced by a radio-frequency current. Topical chemotherapy involves topical applications of caustic or antimetabolite drugs to kill sarcoid cells. Podophyllum and 5-fluorouracil are commonly used for this procedure. Intratumoral chemotherapy involves the use of implants of caustic or antimetabolite drugs within the sarcoids to kill the cells of the tumors. Cisplatin and 5-fluorouracil are commonly used in the implants.

Web site: http://www.delphion.com/details?pn=US06147086__

- **Method for treating patients with sarcoidosis by administering substituted sulfonyl indenyl acetic acids, esters and alcohols**

Inventor(s): Pamukcu; Rifat (Spring House, PA), Piazza; Gary (Doylestown, PA), Skopinska-Rozewska; Ewa (Warsaw, PL)

Assignee(s): Cell Pathways, Inc. (Horsham, PA)

Patent Number: 5,958,982

Date filed: April 17, 1998

Abstract: Substituted indenyl sulfonyl acetic acids, esters and alcohols are useful in the treatment of sarcoidosis.

Excerpt(s): This invention relates to methods for treating sarcoidosis. ... Sarcoidosis is a chronic lung disease of unknown etiology, which is believed to occur when the body's immune system overreacts to an unknown agent. Some authors have noted an association with HLA types B8 and B27 with various manifestations of the disease suggesting that genetic factors may be involved. ... It is often described as incidentall finding as hilar adenopathy on a routine chest x-ray of an asymptomatic individual. The most common clinical findings of sarcoidosis is cough, followed by dyspnea, wheezing and hemoptysis. Auscultation of the lungs is usually unremarkable unless extensive fibrosis is present. Other organs may be involved, with granulomas found in the liver, heart, spleen and bone marrow in nearly half the cases. Eye, skin and salivary glands are involved in about one-third of the cases. Hypercalcemia and hypercalciurea occur in 20-30% of patients and may occasionally result in urolithiasis.

Web site: http://www.delphion.com/details?pn=US05958982__

- **Therapy of sarcoidosis**

  Inventor(s): Wigzell; Hans (Hagersten, SE), Grunewald; Johan (Stockholm, SE), Janson; Carl Harald (Stockholm, SE), Jones; Nancy (Wayland, MA)

  Assignee(s): Avant Immunotherapeutics, Inc. (Needham, MA)

  Patent Number: 5,958,410

  Date filed: November 6, 1995

  Abstract: Sarcoidosis is associated with CD4.sup.+ T lymphocytes which express the T cell receptor V.sub..alpha. 2.3 chain. Thus, a method for diagnosing sarcoidosis is provided which comprises contacting cells of a subject with a first monoclonal antibody, or an antigen-binding fragment or derivative, specific for an epitope of the variable region of the T cell receptor V.sub..alpha. 2.3 chain and detecting the binding of the antibody. Also provided is a method for treating sarcoidosis in which a monoclonal antibody, or an antigen-binding fragment or derivative thereof, specific for an epitope of the variable region of the T cell receptor V.sub..alpha. 2.3 chain is administered. Sarcoidosis is also treated by administering a therapeutically effective amount of a protein or a peptide comprising an amino acid sequence of the variable region of the T cell receptor V.sub..alpha. 2.3 chain, or a functional derivative of the protein or peptide, or an antisense oligonucleotide which is complementary to the T cell receptor V.sub..alpha. 2.3 mRNA.

  Excerpt(s): The present invention in the fields of immunology and medicine relates to methods for diagnosing and treating sarcoidosis based on the presence in the lungs of sarcoidosis patients of T lymphocytes expressing the V.sub.60 2.3 variant of the T cell receptor a chain. Monoclonal antibodies specific for an epitope of the variable region of the T cell receptor V.sub.60 2.3 chain, or epitope-binding fragments or derivatives of the antibody, are useful in diagnostic and therapeutic methods. ... Sarcoidosis is a chronic inflammatory disorder with unknown etiology, characterized by non-caseating granulomas in affected organs, in particular, the lungs, lymph nodes, skin and eyes. The disorder is typically accompanied by nonspecific depression of cell-mediated as well as humoral immune responsiveness, and by polyclonal hypergamma-globulinemia (Siltzbach, L. E., Amer. Rev. Resp. Dis. 97:1-8 (1968); Roberts, C. R. et al., Ann. Intern. Med. 94:73 (1981)). At least 90% of the patients with this multisystem disease have pulmonary manifestations characterized by chronic inflammation, granuloma formation and some cases of pulmonary fibrosis. These processes affect the alveoli, airways and blood vessels resulting in an impairment of normal gas exchange. The inflammatory process precedes the other symptoms of sarcoidosis. ... Certain diseases, in particular those with autoimmune etiologies, are associated with the increase in frequencies of T lymphocytes expressing a particular .alpha. or .beta. TCR V region gene (Hafler, D. A. et al., J. Exp. Med. 167:1313 (1988); Mantegazza, R. et al., Autoimmunity 3:431 (1990)). Such limited or preferential usage of specific TCRs has recently been observed in sarcoidosis (Moller, D. et al., J. Clin. Invest. 82:1183 (1988); Balbi, B. et al., J. Clin. Invest. 85:1353 (1990); Tamura, N. et al., J. Exp. Med. 172:169 (1990)).

Web site: http://www.delphion.com/details?pn=US05958410__

- **Sarcoidosis test**

  Inventor(s): Silverstein; Emanuel (Brooklyn, NY)

  Assignee(s): Research Corporation (New York, NY)

  Patent Number: 4,108,726

  Date filed: July 15, 1976

  Abstract: Serum angiotensin converting enzyme is elevated in many patients with sarcoidosis. A method involving formation of the fluorescent adduct of o-phthaldialdehyde and the histidyl moiety of the L-histidyl-L-leucine product formed by the action of angiotensin converting enzyme on hippuryl-L-histidyl-L-leucine substrate is applicable to determining angiotensin converting enzyme in untreated serum for the diagnosis of sarcoidosis. This method is simple, rapid and highly sensitive, and requires as little as one ul or less of a serum.

  Excerpt(s): This invention relates to serum angiotensin converting enzyme. Serum angiotensin converting enzyme has been observed to be elevated in many patients with sarcoidosis, see Lieberman, J. (1974) A new confirmatory test for sarcoidosis. Serum angiotensin converting enzyme. Effect of steriods and chronic lung disease. Amer. Rev. Resp. Dis. 109, 743 (1974); Silverstein, E., Friedland, J., Lyons, H. and Kitt, M. Serum angiotensin converting enzyme in sarcoidosis. Clin. Res. 23, 352A; Silverstein, E., Friedland, J., Lyons, H. and Gourin, A. Elevated angiotensin converting enzyme activity in non-necrotizing granulomatous lymph nodes in sarcoidosis. Clin. Res. 23, 352A. ... An object of this invention is to provide a method or technique for the diagnosis of sarcoidosis and the like. ... The practice of this invention is based on formation of the fluorescent adduct of o-phthaldialdehyde and the histidyl moiety of the L-histidyl-L-leucine product, see Piquilloud, Y., Reinharz, A., Roth, M. (1970). Studies on angiotensin converting enzyme with different substrates. Biochem. Biophys. Acta. 206, 136-142; Shore, P. A., Burkhalter, A., Cohn, V. H., Jr. (1959). A method for the fluorimetric assay of histamine in tissues. J. Pharm. Exp. Ther. 127, 182; Gregerman, R. I. (1967). Identification of histidyleucine and other histidyl peptides as normal constituents of human urine. Biochem. Med. 1, 151-167, formed from the hippuryl-L-histidyl-L-leucine substrate. This invention is applicable to untreated sera, simple, rapid, and highly sensitive, requiring as little as 1 .mu.l or less of serum and has been applied to the study of large numbers of sera in sarcoidosis, see Silverstein, E., Friedland, J., Lyons, H. and Kitt, M. Serum angiotensin converting enzyme in sarcoidosis. Clin. Res. 23, 352A.

Web site: http://www.delphion.com/details?pn=US04108726__

Patent Applications on Sarcoidosis

As of December 2000, U.S. patent applications are open to public viewing.[25] Applications are patent requests which have yet to be granted (the process to achieve a patent can take several years).

Keeping Current

In order to stay informed about patents and patent applications dealing with sarcoidosis, you can access the U.S. Patent Office archive via the Internet at no cost to you. This archive is available at the following Web address: **http://www.uspto.gov/main/patents.htm**. Under "Services," click on "Search Patents." You will see two broad options: (1) Patent Grants, and (2) Patent Applications. To see a list of granted patents, perform the following steps: Under "Patent Grants," click "Quick Search." Then, type "sarcoidosis" (or

---

[25] This has been a common practice outside the United States prior to December 2000.

synonyms) into the "Term 1" box. After clicking on the search button, scroll down to see the various patents which have been granted to date on sarcoidosis. You can also use this procedure to view pending patent applications concerning sarcoidosis. Simply go back to the following Web address: **http://www.uspto.gov/main/patents.htm**. Under "Services," click on "Search Patents." Select "Quick Search" under "Patent Applications." Then proceed with the steps listed above.

Vocabulary Builder

Abdomen: That portion of the body that lies between the thorax and the pelvis. [NIH]

Antibody: An immunoglobulin molecule that has a specific amino acid sequence by virtue of which it interacts only with the antigen that induced its synthesis in cells of the lymphoid series (especially plasma cells), or with antigen closely related to it. Antibodies are classified according to their ode of action as agglutinins, bacteriolysins, haemolysins, opsonins, precipitins, etc. [EU]

Auscultation: The act of listening for sounds within the body, chiefly for ascertaining the condition of the lungs, heart, pleura, abdomen and other organs, and for the detection of pregnancy. [EU]

Caustic: An escharotic or corrosive agent. Called also cauterant. [EU]

Cisplatin: An inorganic and water-soluble platinum complex. After undergoing hydrolysis, it reacts with DNA to produce both intra and interstrand crosslinks. These crosslinks appear to impair replication and transcription of DNA. The cytotoxicity of cisplatin correlates with cellular arrest in the G2 phase of the cell cycle. [NIH]

Fibroblasts: Connective tissue cells which secrete an extracellular matrix rich in collagen and other macromolecules. [NIH]

Fluorouracil: A pyrimidine analog that acts as an antineoplastic antimetabolite and also has immunosuppressant. It interferes with DNA synthesis by blocking the thymidylate synthetase conversion of deoxyuridylic acid to thymidylic acid. [NIH]

Hemoptysis: Coughing up blood or blood-stained sputum. [NIH]

Histamine: 1H-Imidazole-4-ethanamine. A depressor amine derived by enzymatic decarboxylation of histidine. It is a powerful stimulant of gastric secretion, a constrictor of bronchial smooth muscle, a vasodilator, and also a centrally acting neurotransmitter. [NIH]

Hyperthermia: Abnormally high body temperature, especially that induced for therapeutic purposes. [EU]

Immunotherapy: Manipulation of the host's immune system in treatment of disease. It includes both active and passive immunization as well as immunosuppressive therapy to prevent graft rejection. [NIH]

Leucine: An essential branched-chain amino acid important for hemoglobin formation. [NIH]

Mycobacterium: An organism of the genus Mycobacterium. [EU]

Neoplastic: Pertaining to or like a neoplasm (= any new and abnormal growth); pertaining to neoplasia (= the formation of a neoplasm). [EU]

Nitrogen: An element with the atomic symbol N, atomic number 7, and atomic weight 14. Nitrogen exists as a diatomic gas and makes up about 78% of the earth's atmosphere by volume. It is a constituent of proteins and nucleic acids and found in all living cells. [NIH]

Podophyllum: A genus of poisonous American herbs, family Berberidaceae. The roots yield podophyllotoxins and other pharmacologically important agents. The plant was formerly used as a cholagogue and cathartic. It is different from the European mandrake, mandragora. [NIH]

Substrate: A substance upon which an enzyme acts. [EU]

Wheezing: Breathing with a rasp or whistling sound; a sign of airway constriction or obstruction. [NIH]

CHAPTER 6. BOOKS ON SARCOIDOSIS

Overview

This chapter provides bibliographic book references relating to sarcoidosis. You have many options to locate books on sarcoidosis. The simplest method is to go to your local bookseller and inquire about titles that they have in stock or can special order for you. Some patients, however, feel uncomfortable approaching their local booksellers and prefer online sources (e.g. **www.amazon.com** and **www.bn.com**). In addition to online booksellers, excellent sources for book titles on sarcoidosis include the Combined Health Information Database and the National Library of Medicine. Once you have found a title that interests you, visit your local public or medical library to see if it is available for loan.

Book Summaries: Federal Agencies

The Combined Health Information Database collects various book abstracts from a variety of healthcare institutions and federal agencies. To access these summaries, go directly to the following hyperlink: **http://chid.nih.gov/detail/detail.html**. You will need to use the "Detailed Search" option. To find book summaries, use the drop boxes at the bottom of the search page where "You may refine your search by." Select the dates and language you prefer. For the format option, select "Monograph/Book." Now type "sarcoidosis" (or synonyms) into the "For these words:" box. You will only receive results on books. You should check back periodically with this database which is updated every 3 months. The following is a typical result when searching for books on sarcoidosis:

- **Primer on the Rheumatic Diseases. 11th ed**

Source: Atlanta, GA: Arthritis Foundation. 1997. 529 p.

Contact: Available from Arthritis Foundation. P.O. Box 1616, Alpharetta, GA 30009-1616. (800) 207-8633. Fax (credit card orders only) (770) 442-9742. Website: www.arthritis.org. Price: $39.95 plus shipping and handling.

Summary: This book provides health professionals with a concise, authoritative description of the current science, diagnosis, clinical consequences, and management of the rheumatic diseases. The book begins with chapters on the history of rheumatic diseases and their social and economic consequences. These are followed by chapters that describe the components and structure of the musculoskeletal system; identify the mediators of inflammation, tissue destruction, and repair; and discuss the role of immunity in rheumatic disease. Chapters then focus on evaluating the patient on the basis of medical history, physical examination, and diagnostic tests and present the signs and symptoms of musculoskeletal disorders. Subsequent chapters present an overview of various rheumatic diseases, including rheumatoid arthritis, psoriatic arthritis, seronegative spondyloarthropathies, infectious disorders, rheumatic fever, osteoarthritis, apatites and miscellaneous crystals, calcium pyrophosphate dihydrate crystal deposition, gout, undifferentiated connective tissue syndromes, systemic lupus erythematous, systemic sclerosis and related syndromes, inflammatory and metabolic diseases of muscle, Sjogren's syndrome, vasculitis, polymyalgia rheumatica, and Behcet's disease. Other rheumatic diseases featured include relapsing polychondritis, antiphospholipid syndrome, Adult Still's disease, reflex sympathetic dystrophy and transient regional osteoporosis, neuropathic arthropathy, sarcoidosis, deposition and storage diseases, arthropathies associated with hematologic and malignant disorders and endocrine disease, the amyloidoses, joint neoplasms, musculoskeletal manifestations of hyperlipoproteinemia, musculoskeletal problems in dialysis patients, heritable disorders of connective tissue, hypertrophic osteoarthropathy, bone and joint dysplasias, osteonecrosis, Paget's disease of bone, osteoporosis and metabolic bone diseases, foreign body synovitis, pediatric rheumatic diseases, and miscellaneous syndromes. In addition, the book addresses such issues as rehabilitation of patients who have rheumatic disease, psychosocial factors, patient education, and therapeutic injection of joints and soft tissues. Concluding chapters focus on pharmacological, operative, and questionable methods of treating rheumatic diseases. 5 appendixes, numerous figures, tables, and references.

- **Essential Atlas of Nephrology**

  Source: Philadelphia, PA: Lippincott Williams and Wilkins. 2001. 272 p.

  Contact: Available from Lippincott Williams and Wilkins. P.O. Box 1600, Hagerstown, MD 21741. (800) 638-3030 or (301) 223-2300. Fax (301) 223-2365. Price: $149.00 plus shipping and handling. ISBN: 0781735300.

  Summary: This atlas of nephrology is a compilation of the most important images and topics from a five volume Atlas of Diseases of the Kidney. Eight sections cover disorders of water, electrolytes, and acid base; acute renal (kidney) failure; glomerulonephritis and vasculitis; tubulointerstitial disease; hypertension and the kidney; transplantation as treatment of end stage renal disease (ESRD); dialysis as treatment of ESRD; and systemic diseases and the kidney. Specific topics covered include disorders of sodium balance, potassium metabolism, disorders of acid base balance, the causes and prognosis of acute renal failure (ARF), ARF in the transplanted kidney, nutrition and metabolism in ARF, primary glomerulopathies, vascular disorders, urinary tract infection, reflux and obstructive nephropathy, cystic diseases of the kidney, toxic nephropathies, renal tubular disorders, the kidney in blood pressure regulation, renal parenchymal disease and hypertension (high blood pressure), renovascular hypertension and ischemic nephropathy, adrenal causes of hypertension, insulin resistance and hypertension, pharmacologic treatment of hypertension, histocompatibility testing and organ sharing, transplant rejection and its treatment, posttransplant infections, immunosuppressive therapy and protocols, medical complications of renal transplantation, kidney pancreas transplantation, transplantation in children, recurrent disease in the transplanted kidney, high efficiency and high flux hemodialysis, dialysate composition in hemodialysis and in peritoneal dialysis, dialysis access and recirculation, the dialysis prescription and urea modeling, complications of dialysis, diabetic nephropathy (kidney disease associated with diabetes mellitus), vasculitis, amyloidosis, sickle cell disease, kidney involvement in malignancy (cancer), kidney involvement in tropical diseases, kidney disease in patients with hepatitis and HIV, kidney involvement in sarcoidosis, and kidney disease and hypertension in pregnancy. The information on each topic is provided in table, algorithm, chart, and bulleted format for ease of access. Black and white photographs illustrate many of the chapters; a brief section of color plates concludes the volume.

- **Atlas of Diseases of the Kidney. Volume 4: Systemic Diseases and the Kidney**

  Source: Philadelphia, PA: Current Medicine, Inc. 1999. [234 p.].

Contact: Available from Blackwell Science, Inc. 350 Main Street, Malden, MA 02148. (800) 215-1000 or (781) 388-8250. Fax (781) 388-8270. E-mail: csbooks@blacksci.com. Price: $75.00 plus shipping and handling. ISBN: 0632044373.

Summary: This volume is the fourth in a series of five that make up the Atlas of Diseases of the Kidney, a set that offers educational images including colored photographs, schematics, tables, and algorithms. In Volume 4, the authors describe a number of systemic diseases that may affect the renal parenchyma and other organs. The major emphasis is on the effects on renal function and structure of diseases such as diabetes mellitus, a diverse group of vasculitides (e.g., polyarteritis, Wegener's granulomatosis), amyloidosis, malignancy, viral infections (HIV, hepatitis), collagen vascular diseases, sarcoidosis, and cryoglobulinemia. All the chapters offer diagrams, tables, and illustrations to describe the natural history, clinical manifestations, laboratory findings, pathologic changes, and outcome of entities that affect the function and structure of the kidney. Each chapter features a detailed introduction and lengthy captions for each of the illustrations and diagrams offered. A subject index for Volume 4 and a section of full color plates concludes the book.

The National Library of Medicine Book Index

The National Library of Medicine at the National Institutes of Health has a massive database of books published on healthcare and biomedicine. Go to the following Internet site, **http://locatorplus.gov/**, and then select "Search LOCATORplus." Once you are in the search area, simply type "sarcoidosis" (or synonyms) into the search box, and select "books only." From there, results can be sorted by publication date, author, or relevance. The following was recently catalogued by the National Library of Medicine:[26]

- **Abstracts.** Author: 2nd European Symposium on Sarcoidosis, Berlin, November 3-5, 1976 = Autoreferate / 2. Europäisches Sarkoidose-

---

[26] In addition to LOCATORPlus, in collaboration with authors and publishers, the National Center for Biotechnology Information (NCBI) is adapting biomedical books for the Web. The books may be accessed in two ways: (1) by searching directly using any search term or phrase (in the same way as the bibliographic database PubMed), or (2) by following the links to PubMed abstracts. Each PubMed abstract has a "Books" button that displays a facsimile of the abstract in which some phrases are hypertext links. These phrases are also found in the books available at NCBI. Click on hyperlinked results in the list of books in which the phrase is found. Currently, the majority of the links are between the books and PubMed. In the future, more links will be created between the books and other types of information, such as gene and protein sequences and macromolecular structures. See **http://www.ncbi.nlm.nih.gov/entrez/query.fcgi?db=Books.**

Symposium, Berlin, 3.-5. November 1976; Year: 1976; [East Germany: s.n., 1976?]

- **Angiotensin converting enzyme and sarcoidosis.** Author: by Carola Grönhagen-Riska; Year: 1980; Helsinki: [s.n.], 1980; ISBN: 9519927204

- **Clinical and biochemical aspects of sarcoidosis: with special reference to angiotensin-converting enzyme (ACE).** Author: by Frode K. Rømer; Year: 1984; Stockholm, Sweden: Distributed by Almqvist & Wiksell Periodical Co., 1984

- **Eighth International Conference on Sarcoidosis and other Granulomatous Diseases.** Author: editors, W. Jones Williams, Brian H. Davies; Year: 1980; Cardiff, Wales: Alpha Omega Pub., c1980; ISBN: 0900663103
  http://www.amazon.com/exec/obidos/ASIN/0900663103/icongroupin terna

- **Evaluative report on completed contracts awarded in response to RFP NHLI 74-7: developments of an in vitro diagnostic test for sarcoidosis, December 1978.** Author: issued by Division of Lung Diseases, National Heart, Lung, and Blood Institute; Year: 1979; [Bethesda, Md.]: U. S. Dept. of Health, Education, and Welfare, Public Health Service, National Institutes of Health, 1979

- **Immunological studies in sarcoidosis.** Author: by Eva Hedfors; Year: 1974; Stockholm: Repro Print, 1974

- **Lymphocyte transformation in sarcoidosis.** Author: by Maija Horsmanheimo; Year: 1973; Helsinki: [s.n.], 1973

- **Ophthalmic changes in sarcoidosis.** Author: by Anni Karma; Year: 1979; Copenhagen: Seriptor, 1979

- **Sarcoidosis: January 1974 through May 1976: 361 citations in English or with English abstract.** Author: prepared by Geraldine D. Nowak; Year: 1976; [Bethesda, Md.]: U. S. Dept. of Health, Education, and Welfare, Public Health Service, National Institutes of Health, [1976]

- **Sarcoidosis: January 1982 through September 1984: 353 citations.** Author: prepared by Charlotte Kenton; Year: 1984; [Bethesda, Md.]: U.S. Dept. of Health and Human Services, Public Health Service, National Institutes of Health, 1984

- **Sarcoidosis: proceedings of the International Symposium on Sarcoidosis held November 14-16, 1979.** Author: edited by Riichiro Mikami, Yutaka Hosoda; Year: 1981; [Tokyo]: University of Tokyo Press, c1981

- **Sarcoidosis: resource guide and directory: a medical mystery uncovered, facts, information, and helplines.** Author: by Sandra

Conroy; Year: 1991; Piscataway, N.J.: PC Publications, c1991; ISBN: 0963122258
http://www.amazon.com/exec/obidos/ASIN/0963122258/icongroupin terna

- **Sarcoidosis and other granulomatous diseases of the lung.** Author: edited by Barry L. Fanburg; Year: 1983; New York: Dekker, c1983; ISBN: 0824718666
http://www.amazon.com/exec/obidos/ASIN/0824718666/icongroupin terna

- **Sarcoidosis and other granulomatous disorders: ninth international conference, Paris, August 31-September 4, 1981.** Author: editors, J. Chrétien, J. Marsac, J.C. Saltiel; Year: 1983; Paris; New York: Pergamon, c1983; ISBN: 0080270883
http://www.amazon.com/exec/obidos/ASIN/0080270883/icongroupin terna

- **Sarcoidosis and other granulomatous disorders: proceedings of the XI World Congress on Sarcoidosis and Other Granulomatous Disorders, Milan, 6-11 September 1987.** Author: editors, Carlo Grassi, Gianfranco Rizzato, Ernesto Pozzi; Year: 1988; Amsterdam; New York: Excerpta Medica; New York, NY, USA: Sole distributors for the USA and Canada, Elsevier Science Pub. Co., 1988; ISBN: 044480983X (U.S.)
http://www.amazon.com/exec/obidos/ASIN/044480983X/icongroupi nterna

- **Sarcoidosis and other granulomatous disorders.** Author: edited by D. Geraint James; Year: 1994; New York: M. Dekker, c1994; ISBN: 0824791266 (alk. paper)
http://www.amazon.com/exec/obidos/ASIN/0824791266/icongroupin terna

- **Sarcoidosis and other granulomatous disorders.** Author: D. Geraint James and W. Jones Williams; Year: 1985; Philadelphia: Saunders, 1985; ISBN: 0721610447
http://www.amazon.com/exec/obidos/ASIN/0721610447/icongroupin terna

- **Sarcoidosis of the respiratory system.** Author: guest editor, D. Geraint James; Year: 1986; New York: Thieme, [c1986]

- **Sarcoidosis.** Author: Takateru Izumi, guest editor; Year: 1986; Philadelphia: Lippincott, c1986

- **Sarcoidosis.** Author: J.G. Scadding and D.N. Mitchell; Year: 1985; London: Chapman and Hall, 1985; ISBN: 0412217600
http://www.amazon.com/exec/obidos/ASIN/0412217600/icongroupin terna

- **Sarcoidosis.** Author: edited by Jack Lieberman; Year: 1985; Orlando: Grune & Stratton, c1985; ISBN: 0808917285
  http://www.amazon.com/exec/obidos/ASIN/0808917285/icongroupin
  terna

- **Sarcoidosis: a serial roentgenographic study.** Author: Holt, Allen H., 1924-; Year: 1955; [Minneapolis] 1955

- **Sarcoidosis; a clinical approach.** Author: Sharma, Om P; Year: 1975; Springfield, Ill., Thomas [c1975]; ISBN: 039803303X
  http://www.amazon.com/exec/obidos/ASIN/039803303X/icongroupi
  nterna

- **Sarcoidosis--clinical management.** Author: Om P. Sharma; Year: 1984; London; Boston: Butterworths, 1984; ISBN: 0407003266
  http://www.amazon.com/exec/obidos/ASIN/0407003266/icongroupin
  terna

- **Seventh International Conference on Sarcoidosis and other Granulomatous Disorders.** Author: edited by Louis E. Siltzbach; Year: 1976; New York: New York Academy of Sciences, 1976; ISBN: 0890720576
  http://www.amazon.com/exec/obidos/ASIN/0890720576/icongroupin
  terna

- **Tenth International Conference on Sarcoidosis and Other Granulomatous Disorders.** Author: edited by Carol Johnson Johns; Year: 1986; New York, N.Y.: New York Academy of Sciences, 1986; ISBN: 089766325X
  http://www.amazon.com/exec/obidos/ASIN/089766325X/icongroupi
  nterna

Chapters on Sarcoidosis

Frequently, sarcoidosis will be discussed within a book, perhaps within a specific chapter. In order to find chapters that are specifically dealing with sarcoidosis, an excellent source of abstracts is the Combined Health Information Database. You will need to limit your search to book chapters and sarcoidosis using the "Detailed Search" option. Go directly to the following hyperlink: **http://chid.nih.gov/detail/detail.html**. To find book chapters, use the drop boxes at the bottom of the search page where "You may refine your search by." Select the dates and language you prefer, and the format option "Book Chapter." By making these selections and typing in "sarcoidosis" (or synonyms) into the "For these words:" box, you will only receive results on chapters in books. The following is a typical result when searching for book chapters on sarcoidosis:

- **Sarcoidosis**

   Source: in Maddison, P.J.; et al., Eds. Oxford Textbook of Rheumatology. Volume 2. New York, NY: Oxford University Press, Inc. 1993. p. 928-933.

   Contact: Available from Oxford University Press, Inc., New York, NY.

   Summary: This chapter for health professionals presents an overview of sarcoidosis. This multisystem disease is characterized by multiple, noncaseating granulomata in involved tissues. The etiology, pathology, and epidemiology of sarcoidosis are discussed. The general clinical features of acute and chronic sarcoidosis are highlighted. Data on the outcome of various laboratory investigations for sarcoidosis are presented, focusing on results of routine investigations, serial measurements of angiotensin-converting enzyme, the Kveim test, diagnostic imaging, histological studies, and bronchonalveolar lavage. Musculoskeletal manifestations of sarcoidosis are described, including joint, bone, and muscle disease. Treatment options for sarcoidosis are highlighted. 31 references, 9 figures, and 1 table.

- **Lip Lesions**

   Source: in Scully, C. and Cawson, R.A. Oral Disease: Colour Guide. 2nd ed. Edinburgh, Scotland: Churchill Livingstone. 1999. p. 1-22.

   Contact: Available from W.B. Saunders Company, A Harcourt Health Sciences Company. Book Order Fulfillment Department, 11830 Westline Industrial Drive, St Louis, MO 63146-9988. (800) 545-2522. Fax (800) 568-5136. E-mail: wbsbcs@harcourt.com. Website: www.wbsaunders.com. Price: $19.95 plus shipping and handling. ISBN: 044306170X.

   Summary: This chapter on lip lesions is from a book that is intended as an aid to oral medicine and the diagnosis and treatment of oral disease. The chapter includes 24 full color photographs of lip lesions, with textual information accompanying them. Conditions covered are: herpes labialis, herpes zoster (shingles), impetigo contagiosa, primary syphilis (Hunterian or hard chancre), pyogenic granuloma, carcinoma (cancer), erythema multiforme, leukemia, discoid lupus erythematosus (DLE), lichen planus, angular stomatitis, cracked lip, actinic burns, allergic angioedema, hereditary angioedema, oral Crohn's disease, sarcoidosis, nevi, Peutz-Jeghers syndrome, mucocele, and Sturge-Weber syndrome (encephalotrigeminal angiomatosis). For each condition, the text briefly covers incidence and etiology, clinical features, diagnosis and diagnostic tests, and treatment options.

- **Major Salivary Gland Disease**

  Source: in Scully, C. and Cawson, R.A. Oral Disease: Colour Guide. 2nd ed. Edinburgh, Scotland: Churchill Livingstone. 1999. p. 135-144.

  Contact: Available from W.B. Saunders Company, A Harcourt Health Sciences Company. Book Order Fulfillment Department, 11830 Westline Industrial Drive, St Louis, MO 63146-9988. (800) 545-2522. Fax (800) 568-5136. E-mail: wbsbcs@harcourt.com. Website: www.wbsaunders.com. Price: $19.95 plus shipping and handling. ISBN: 044306170X.

  Summary: This chapter on major salivary gland diseases is from a book that is intended as an aid to oral medicine and the diagnosis and treatment of oral disease. The chapter includes 10 full color photographs of salivary gland diseases, with textual information accompanying them. Conditions covered are: mumps (acute viral parotitis), acute bacterial (ascending) parotitis, salivary obstruction, sarcoidosis, Sjogren syndrome, dry mouth, sialosis (swelling of the parotid glands), and salivary gland neoplasms. For each condition, the text briefly covers incidence and etiology, clinical features, diagnosis and diagnostic tests, and treatment options.

- **Salivary Gland Disorders**

  Source: in Wray, D., et al. Textbook of General and Oral Medicine. Edinburgh, Scotland: Churchill Livingstone. 1999. p. 279-292.

  Contact: Available from Harcourt Health Sciences. 11830 Westline Industrial Drive, St. Louis, MO 63146. (800) 325-4177. Fax (800) 874-6418. Website: www.harcourthealth.com. Price: $50.00 plus shipping and handling. ISBN: 0443051895.

  Summary: Disease processes involving the salivary glands may present as swellings, too little saliva (xerostomia), too much saliva (sialorrhea or ptyalism), or other conditions such as necrotizing sialometaplasia or salivary fistula. This chapter on salivary gland disorders is from an undergraduate dentistry textbook that covers both general medicine and surgery, and oral medicine, emphasizing the overlap between them. The authors begin the chapter with a discussion of the proper diagnosis of salivary gland disease, including the use of salivary flow rates (sialometry), sialochemistry (analysis of the constituents of saliva), plain radiography, sialography, scintiscanning, and salivary gland biopsy. The authors then discuss salivary gland swellings, including that caused by bacterial sialadenitis, and recurrent parotitis of childhood; duct obstruction; systemic infections, including mumps and HIV parotitis; Sjogren's syndrome; sarcoidosis; sialosis; drugs; and neoplasms (including cancer). The authors then discuss xerostomia (dry mouth) and its developmental and iatrogenic causes. Clinical points to remember are highlighted in text boxes. 13 figures. 11 tables.

- **Respiratory Disorders**

Source: in Scully, C. and Cawson, R.A. Medical Problems in Dentistry. 4th ed. Woburn, MA: Butterworth-Heinemann. 1998. p. 154-172.

Contact: Available from Butterworth-Heinemann. 225 Wildwood Avenue, Woburn, MA 01801-2041. (800) 366-2665 or (781) 904-2500. Fax (800) 446-6520 or (781) 933-6333. E-mail: orders@bhusa.com. Website: www.bh.com. Price: $110.00. ISBN: 0723610568.

Summary: Respiratory disorders are common and may significantly affect dental treatment, especially general anesthesia. Respiratory diseases are often also a contraindication to opioids, benzodiazepines and other respiratory depressants. This chapter on respiratory disorders is from a text that covers the general medical and surgical conditions relevant to the oral health care sciences. Topics include upper respiratory tract viral infections, sinusitis, lower respiratory tract infections, pulmonary tuberculosis, Legionnaire's disease (legionellosis), lung abscess, bronchiectasis, cystic fibrosis, chronic obstructive airways diseases, asthma, bronchogenic carcinoma (lung cancer), occupational lung disease, sarcoidosis, postoperative respiratory complications (including aspiration of gastric contents), obstructive sleep apnea syndrome, and respiratory distress syndromes (RDS). For each disease, the authors discuss general aspects, diagnosis and management issues, dental aspects, and patient care strategies. The chapter includes a summary of the points covered. 1 figure. 5 tables. 51 references.

- **Salivary Glands**

Source: in Ballenger, J.J.; Snow, J.B., Jr., eds. Otorhinolaryngology: Head and Neck Surgery. 15th ed. Baltimore, MD: Williams and Wilkins. 1996. p. 390-400.

Contact: Available from Williams and Wilkins. P.O. Box 64786, Baltimore, MD 21264-4786. (800) 638-0672; Fax (800) 447-8438. Price: $179.00 plus shipping and handling. ISBN: 0683003151.

Summary: This chapter, from a medical text on otorhinolaryngology, considers the anatomy, physiology, and major disease processes of the major and minor salivary glands. Pathology topics covered include hormonal and metabolic disorders; endocrine disorders; drug effects; inflammatory disorders; and systemic inflammatory diseases affecting the salivary glands, including viral infections, Sjogren's syndrome, benign lymphoepithelial lesion, human immunodeficiency virus (HIV), sarcoidosis, and Wegener's granulomatosis. Additional sections consider granulomatous diseases; inflammatory disease isolated to the salivary glands; benign parotid neoplasms; malignant neoplasms; and imaging techniques used for the salivary glands, including contrast sialography, computed tomography (CT), and magnetic resonance imaging. 1 figure. 1 table. 25 references.

- **Chapter 184: Sarcoidosis of the Skin**

Source: in Freedberg, I.M., et al., eds. Fitzpatrick's Dermatology in General Medicine. 5th ed., Vol. 2. New York, NY: McGraw-Hill. 1999. p. 2099-2106.

Contact: Available from McGraw-Hill Customer Services. P.O. Box 548, Blacklick, OH 43004-0548. (800) 262-4729 or (877) 833-5524. Fax (614) 759-3749 or (614) 759-3641. E-mail: customer.service@mcgraw-hill.com. Price: $395.00 plus shipping and handling. ISBN: 0070219435.

Summary: This chapter provides health professionals with information on the clinical features, pathogenesis, laboratory findings, immunology, diagnosis, and treatment of sarcoidosis of the skin. Skin lesions occur in about one-fourth of patients who have sarcoidosis. The lesions of sarcoidosis are lupus pernio, plaques, and maculopapular eruptions. Lupus pernio, the most characteristic of all sarcoid skin lesions, is a chronic, violaceous, indurated skin lesion. Skin plaques are purplish, elevated, indurated patches usually located on the limbs, face, back, and buttocks. Papular eruptions are the most common skin manifestation of sarcoidosis in African Americans. Other skin changes include subcutaneous nodules; scarring from atrophy, trauma, surgery, or venipuncture; and erythema nodosum. The clinical manifestations of sarcoidosis depend on age, race, duration of the illness, site and extent of tissue involvement, and activity of the granulomatous process. Patients with sarcoidosis may complain of various nonspecific symptoms, or they may experience respiratory symptoms, chest radiographic abnormalities, lung function abnormalities, granulomatous uveitis, enlarged peripheral lymph nodes, and spleen enlargement. In addition, the gastrointestinal tract, heart, musculosketelal system, kidneys, salivary glands, upper respiratory tract, endocrine glands, and nervous system may be involved. Laboratory findings include hypercalcemia and increased serum angiotensin-converting enzyme in about 60 percent of patients. Immunologic features include depression of cutaneous delayed-type hypersensitivity reactions, lymphopenia, and expansion of the T lymphocytes in bronchoalveolar lavage fluid. Diagnosis is based on a compatible clinical or radiographic picture, histologic evidence of noncaseating granulomas, and negative special stains and cultures for other entities. Therapeutic options include glucocorticoids, antimalarials, immunosuppressive drugs, and cosmetic surgery. 6 figures and 14 references.

Directories

In addition to the references and resources discussed earlier in this chapter, a number of directories relating to sarcoidosis have been published that consolidate information across various sources. These too might be useful in gaining access to additional guidance on sarcoidosis. The Combined Health Information Database lists the following, which you may wish to consult in your local medical library:[27]

- **1998-1999 Complete Directory for People with Rare Disorders**

  Source: Lakeville, CT: Grey House Publishing, Inc. 1998. 726 p.

  Contact: Available from Grey House Publishing, Inc. Pocket Knife Square, Lakeville, CT 06039. (860) 435-0868. Fax (860) 435-0867. PRICE: $190.00. ISBN: 0939300982.

  Summary: This directory, from the National Organization for Rare Disorders (NORD) provides a wealth of information on diseases and organizations. The directory offers four sections: disease descriptions, disease specific organizations, umbrella organizations, and government agencies. In the first section, the directory includes descriptions of 1,102 rare diseases in alphabetical order. Each entry defines the disorder, then refers readers to the organizations that might be of interest. Diseases related to digestive diseases include achalasia, Addison's disease, Alagille syndrome, Barrett's esophagus, Budd Chiari syndrome, Caroli disease, celiac sprue, cholangitis, cholecystitis, cirrhosis, colitis, Crohn's disease, Cushing syndrome, cystic fibrosis, diverticulitis, Dubin Johnson syndrome, fructose intolerance, galactosemia, gastritis, gastroesophageal reflux, hepatitis, Hirschprung's disease, Hurler syndrome, imperforate anus, irritable bowel syndrome, jejunal atresia, Korsakoff's syndrome, lipodystrophy, maple syrup urine disease, Morquio syndrome, polyposis,

---

[27] You will need to limit your search to "Directories" and sarcoidosis using the "Detailed Search" option. Go directly to the following hyperlink: **http://chid.nih.gov/detail/detail.html**. To find directories, use the drop boxes at the bottom of the search page where "You may refine your search by". For publication date, select "All Years", select language and the format option "Directory". By making these selections and typing in "sarcoidosis" (or synonyms) into the "For these words:" box, you will only receive results on directories dealing with sarcoidosis. You should check back periodically with this database as it is updated every three months.

porphyria, proctitis, prune belly syndrome, sarcoidosis, Stevens Johnson syndrome, Tropical sprue, tyrosinemia, valinemia, vitamin E deficiency, Whipple's disease, Wilson's disease, and Zollinger Ellison syndrome. Each of the 445 organizations listed in the second section is associated with a specific disease or group of diseases. In addition to contact information, there is a descriptive paragraph about the organization and its primary goals and program activities. Entries include materials published by the organization as well as the diseases the organizations cover, which refer readers to Section I. The third section lists 444 organizations that are more general in nature, serving a wide range of diseases (for example, the American Liver Foundation). The final section describes 74 agencies that are important federal government contacts that serve the diverse needs of individuals with rare disorders. A name and key word index concludes the volume.

General Home References

In addition to references for sarcoidosis, you may want a general home medical guide that spans all aspects of home healthcare. The following list is a recent sample of such guides (sorted alphabetically by title; hyperlinks provide rankings, information, and reviews at Amazon.com):

- **Anatomica : The Complete Home Medical Reference** by Peter Forrestal (Editor); Hardcover (2000), Book Sales; ISBN: 1740480309; http://www.amazon.com/exec/obidos/ASIN/1740480309/icongroupinterna

- **The Breathing Disorders Sourcebook** by Francis V. Adams, M.D.; Paperback - 240 pages (November 1998), McGraw Hill - NTC; ISBN: 073730006X; http://www.amazon.com/exec/obidos/ASIN/073730006X/icongroupinterna

- **The HarperCollins Illustrated Medical Dictionary : The Complete Home Medical Dictionary** by Ida G. Dox, et al; Paperback - 656 pages 4th edition (2001), Harper Resource; ISBN: 0062736469; http://www.amazon.com/exec/obidos/ASIN/0062736469/icongroupinterna

- **The Merck Manual of Medical Information: Home Edition (Merck Manual of Medical Information Home Edition (Trade Paper)** by Robert Berkow (Editor), Mark H. Beers, M.D. (Editor); Paperback - 1536 pages (2000), Pocket Books; ISBN: 0671027263; http://www.amazon.com/exec/obidos/ASIN/0671027263/icongroupinterna

- **Stedman's Cardiovascular & Pulmonary Words: Includes Respiratory;** Paperback - 888 pages, 3rd edition (June 15, 2001), Lippincott, Williams &

Wilkins Publishers; ISBN: 0781730562;
http://www.amazon.com/exec/obidos/ASIN/0781730562/icongroupinterna

Vocabulary Builder

Abscess: A localized collection of pus caused by suppuration buried in tissues, organs, or confined spaces. [EU]

Algorithms: A procedure consisting of a sequence of algebraic formulas and/or logical steps to calculate or determine a given task. [NIH]

Anemia: A reduction in the number of circulating erythrocytes or in the quantity of hemoglobin. [NIH]

Anesthesia: A state characterized by loss of feeling or sensation. This depression of nerve function is usually the result of pharmacologic action and is induced to allow performance of surgery or other painful procedures. [NIH]

Angioedema: A vascular reaction involving the deep dermis or subcutaneous or submucal tissues, representing localized edema caused by dilatation and increased permeability of the capillaries, and characterized by development of giant wheals. [EU]

Antibiotics: Substances produced by microorganisms that can inhibit or suppress the growth of other microorganisms. [NIH]

Antineoplastic: Inhibiting or preventing the development of neoplasms, checking the maturation and proliferation of malignant cells. [EU]

Apnea: A transient absence of spontaneous respiration. [NIH]

Arthropathy: Any joint disease. [EU]

Aspiration: The act of inhaling. [EU]

Atrophy: A wasting away; a diminution in the size of a cell, tissue, organ, or part. [EU]

Audiology: The study of hearing and hearing impairment. [NIH]

Barotrauma: Injury following pressure changes; includes injury to the eustachian tube, ear drum, lung and stomach. [NIH]

Benign: Not malignant; not recurrent; favourable for recovery. [EU]

Benzodiazepines: A two-ring heterocyclic compound consisting of a benzene ring fused to a diazepine ring. Permitted is any degree of hydrogenation, any substituents and any H-isomer. [NIH]

Biochemical: Relating to biochemistry; characterized by, produced by, or involving chemical reactions in living organisms. [EU]

Bronchiectasis: Chronic dilatation of the bronchi marked by fetid breath and paroxysmal coughing, with the expectoration of mucopurulent matter. It may effect the tube uniformly (cylindric b.), or occur in irregular pockets (sacculated b.) or the dilated tubes may have terminal bulbous enlargements (fusiform b.). [EU]

Cardiovascular: Pertaining to the heart and blood vessels. [EU]

Chancre: The primary sore of syphilis, a painless indurated, eroded papule, occurring at the site of entry of the infection. [NIH]

Cheilitis: Inflammation of the lips. It is of various etiologies and degrees of pathology. [NIH]

Cholangitis: Inflammation of a bile duct. [EU]

Cholecystitis: Inflammation of the gallbladder, caused primarily by gallstones. Gallbladder disease occurs most often in obese women older than 40 years of age. [NIH]

Cochlear: Of or pertaining to the cochlea. [EU]

Collagen: The protein substance of the white fibres (collagenous fibres) of skin, tendon, bone, cartilage, and all other connective tissue; composed of molecules of tropocollagen (q.v.), it is converted into gelatin by boiling. collagenous pertaining to collagen; forming or producing collagen. [EU]

Cryoglobulinemia: A condition characterized by the presence of abnormal or abnormal quantities of cryoglobulins in the blood. They are precipitated into the microvasculature on exposure to cold and cause restricted blood flow in exposed areas. [NIH]

Dermatosis: Any skin disease, especially one not characterized by inflammation. [EU]

Diverticulitis: Inflammation of a diverticulum, especially inflammation related to colonic diverticula, which may undergo perforation with abscess formation. Sometimes called left-sided or L-sides appendicitis. [EU]

Dysplasia: Abnormal development or growth. [NIH]

Dystrophy: Any disorder arising from defective or faulty nutrition, especially the muscular dystrophies. [EU]

Electrolyte: A substance that dissociates into ions when fused or in solution, and thus becomes capable of conducting electricity; an ionic solute. [EU]

Erythromycin: A bacteriostatic antibiotic substance produced by Streptomyces erythreus. Erythromycin A is considered its major active component. In sensitive organisms, it inhibits protein synthesis by binding to 50S ribosomal subunits. This binding process inhibits peptidyl transferase activity and interferes with translocation of amino acids during translation and assembly of proteins. [NIH]

Gastritis: Inflammation of the stomach. [EU]

Gastrointestinal: Pertaining to or communicating with the stomach and intestine, as a gastrointestinal fistula. [EU]

Gingivitis: Inflammation of the gingivae. Gingivitis associated with bony changes is referred to as periodontitis. Called also oulitis and ulitis. [EU]

Gluten: The protein of wheat and other grains which gives to the dough its tough elastic character. [EU]

Gout: Hereditary metabolic disorder characterized by recurrent acute arthritis, hyperuricemia and deposition of sodium urate in and around the joints, sometimes with formation of uric acid calculi. [NIH]

Herpes: Any inflammatory skin disease caused by a herpesvirus and characterized by the formation of clusters of small vesicles. When used alone, the term may refer to herpes simplex or to herpes zoster. [EU]

Histiocytosis: General term for the abnormal appearance of histiocytes in the blood. Based on the pathological features of the cells involved rather than on clinical findings, the histiocytic diseases are subdivided into three groups: histiocytosis, langerhans cell; histiocytosis, non-langerhans cell; and histiocytic disorders, malignant. [NIH]

Histocompatibility: The degree of antigenic similarity between the tissues of different individuals, which determines the acceptance or rejection of allografts. [NIH]

Hyperlipoproteinemia: Metabolic disease characterized by elevated plasma cholesterol and/or triglyceride levels. The inherited form is attributed to a single gene mechanism. [NIH]

Hyperostosis: Hypertrophy of bone; exostosis. [EU]

Hypertension: High blood pressure (i.e., abnormally high blood pressure tension involving systolic and/or diastolic levels). The Sixth Report of the Joint National Committee on Prevention, Detection, Evaluation, and Treatment of High Blood Pressure defines hypertension as a systolic blood pressure of 140 mm Hg or greater, a diastolic blood pressure of 90 mm Hg or greater, or taking hypertensive medication. The cause may be adrenal, benign, essential, Goldblatt's, idiopathic, malignant PATE, portal, postpartum, primary, pulmonary, renal or renovascular. [NIH]

Hyperthyroidism: 1. excessive functional activity of the thyroid gland. 2. the abnormal condition resulting from hyperthyroidism marked by increased metabolic rate, enlargement of the thyroid gland, rapid heart rate, high blood pressure, and various secondary symptoms. [EU]

Hypothyroidism: Deficiency of thyroid activity. In adults, it is most common in women and is characterized by decrease in basal metabolic rate, tiredness and lethargy, sensitivity to cold, and menstrual disturbances. If untreated, it progresses to full-blown myxoedema. In infants, severe hypothyroidism leads to cretinism. In juveniles, the manifestations are intermediate, with less severe mental and developmental retardation and only mild symptoms of the adult form. When due to pituitary deficiency of thyrotropin secretion it is called secondary hypothyroidism. [EU]

Iatrogenic: Resulting from the activity of physicians. Originally applied to disorders induced in the patient by autosuggestion based on the physician's examination, manner, or discussion, the term is now applied to any adverse condition in a patient occurring as the result of treatment by a physician or surgeon, especially to infections acquired by the patient during the course of treatment. [EU]

Impetigo: A common superficial bacterial infection caused by staphylococcus aureus or group A beta-hemolytic streptococci. Characteristics include pustular lesions that rupture and discharge a thin, amber-colored fluid that dries and forms a crust. This condition is commonly located on the face, especially about the mouth and nose. [NIH]

Insulin: A protein hormone secreted by beta cells of the pancreas. Insulin plays a major role in the regulation of glucose metabolism, generally promoting the cellular utilization of glucose. It is also an important regulator of protein and lipid metabolism. Insulin is used as a drug to control insulin-dependent diabetes mellitus. [NIH]

Labyrinthitis: Inflammation of the inner ear. [NIH]

Legionellosis: Infections with bacteria of the genus legionella. [NIH]

Lipodystrophy: 1. any disturbance of fat metabolism. 2. a group of conditions due to defective metabolism of fat, resulting in the absence of subcutaneous fat, which may be congenital or acquired and partial or total. Called also lipoatrophy and lipodystrophia. [EU]

Maculopapular: Both macular and papular, as an eruption consisting of both macules and papules; sometimes erroneously used to designate a papule that is only slightly elevated. [EU]

Masticatory: 1. subserving or pertaining to mastication; affecting the muscles of mastication. 2. a remedy to be chewed but not swallowed. [EU]

Meningitis: Inflammation of the meninges. When it affects the dura mater, the disease is termed pachymeningitis; when the arachnoid and pia mater are involved, it is called leptomeningitis, or meningitis proper. [EU]

Mucus: A thick fluid produced by the lining of some organs of the body. [NIH]

Mycoplasma: A genus of gram-negative, facultatively anaerobic bacteria bounded by a plasma membrane only. Its organisms are parasites and pathogens, found on the mucous membranes of humans, animals, and birds. [NIH]

Myeloma: A tumour composed of cells of the type normally found in the bone marrow. [EU]

Neoplasms: New abnormal growth of tissue. Malignant neoplasms show a greater degree of anaplasia and have the properties of invasion and metastasis, compared to benign neoplasms. [NIH]

Orofacial: Of or relating to the mouth and face. [EU]

Osteoarthritis: Noninflammatory degenerative joint disease occurring chiefly in older persons, characterized by degeneration of the articular cartilage, hypertrophy of bone at the margins, and changes in the synovial membrane. It is accompanied by pain and stiffness. [NIH]

Osteodystrophy: Defective bone formation. [EU]

Osteogenesis: The histogenesis of bone including ossification. It occurs continuously but particularly in the embryo and child and during fracture repair. [NIH]

Osteonecrosis: Death of a bone or part of a bone, either atraumatic or posttraumatic. [NIH]

Osteopetrosis: Excessive formation of dense trabecular bone leading to pathological fractures, osteitis, splenomegaly with infarct, anemia, and extramedullary hemopoiesis. [NIH]

Osteoporosis: Reduction in the amount of bone mass, leading to fractures after minimal trauma. [EU]

Otolaryngology: A surgical specialty concerned with the study and treatment of disorders of the ear, nose, and throat. [NIH]

Otorhinolaryngology: That branch of medicine concerned with medical and surgical treatment of the head and neck, including the ears, nose and throat. [EU]

Otosclerosis: A pathological condition of the bony labyrinth of the ear, in which there is formation of spongy bone (otospongiosis), especially in front of and posterior to the footplate of the stapes; it may cause bony ankylosis of the stapes, resulting in conductive hearing loss. Cochlear otosclerosis may also develop, resulting in sensorineural hearing loss. [EU]

Pacemaker: An object or substance that influences the rate at which a certain phenomenon occurs; often used alone to indicate the natural cardiac pacemaker or an artificial cardiac pacemaker. In biochemistry, a substance whose rate of reaction sets the pace for a series of interrelated reactions. [EU]

Pancreas: A mixed exocrine and endocrine gland situated transversely across the posterior abdominal wall in the epigastric and hypochondriac regions. The endocrine portion is comprised of the islets of langerhans, while the exocrine portion is a compound acinar gland that secretes digestive enzymes. [NIH]

Panniculitis: An inflammatory reaction of the subcutaneous fat, which may involve the connective tissue septa between the fat lobes, the septa lobules and vessels, or the fat lobules, characterized by the development of single or multiple cutaneous nodules. [EU]

Parotitis: Inflammation of the parotid gland. Called also parotiditis. [EU]

Pathologic: 1. indicative of or caused by a morbid condition. 2. pertaining to pathology (= branch of medicine that treats the essential nature of the disease, especially the structural and functional changes in tissues and organs of the body caused by the disease). [EU]

Perineal: Pertaining to the perineum. [EU]

Postoperative: Occurring after a surgical operation. [EU]

Potassium: An element that is in the alkali group of metals. It has an atomic symbol K, atomic number 19, and atomic weight 39.10. It is the chief cation in the intracellular fluid of muscle and other cells. Potassium ion is a strong electrolyte and it plays a significant role in the regulation of fluid volume and maintenance of the water-electrolyte balance. [NIH]

Preoperative: Preceding an operation. [EU]

Presbycusis: Progressive bilateral loss of hearing that occurs in the aged. Syn: senile deafness. [NIH]

Proctitis: Inflammation of the rectum. [EU]

Pyoderma: Any purulent skin disease. Called also pyodermia. [EU]

Pyogenic: Producing pus; pyopoietic (= liquid inflammation product made up of cells and a thin fluid called liquor puris). [EU]

Radiography: The making of film records (radiographs) of internal structures of the body by passage of x-rays or gamma rays through the body to act on specially sensitized film. [EU]

Reflex: 1; reflected. 2. a reflected action or movement; the sum total of any particular involuntary activity. [EU]

Reflux: A backward or return flow. [EU]

Renovascular: Of or pertaining to the blood vessels of the kidneys. [EU]

Rheumatology: A subspecialty of internal medicine concerned with the study of inflammatory or degenerative processes and metabolic derangement of connective tissue structures which pertain to a variety of musculoskeletal disorders, such as arthritis. [NIH]

Riboflavin: Nutritional factor found in milk, eggs, malted barley, liver, kidney, heart, and leafy vegetables. The richest natural source is yeast. It occurs in the free form only in the retina of the eye, in whey, and in urine; its principal forms in tissues and cells are as FMN and FAD. [NIH]

Rubella: An acute, usually benign, infectious disease caused by a togavirus and most often affecting children and nonimmune young adults, in which the virus enters the respiratory tract via droplet nuclei and spreads to the lymphatic system. It is characterized by a slight cold, sore throat, and fever, followed by enlargement of the postauricular, suboccipital, and cervical lymph nodes, and the appearances of a fine pink rash that begins on the head and spreads to become generalized. Called also German measles, roetln, röteln, and three-day measles, and rubeola in French and Spanish. [EU]

Sialography: Radiography of the salivary glands or ducts following injection of contrast medium. [NIH]

Sialorrhea: Increased salivary flow. [NIH]

Sinusitis: Inflammation of a sinus. The condition may be purulent or nonpurulent, acute or chronic. Depending on the site of involvement it is known as ethmoid, frontal, maxillary, or sphenoid sinusitis. [EU]

Spondylitis: Inflammation of the vertebrae. [EU]

Stomatitis: Inflammation of the oral mucosa, due to local or systemic factors which may involve the buccal and labial mucosa, palate, tongue, floor of the mouth, and the gingivae. [EU]

Synovitis: Inflammation of a synovial membrane. It is usually painful, particularly on motion, and is characterized by a fluctuating swelling due to effusion within a synovial sac. Synovitis is qualified as fibrinous, gonorrhoeal, hyperplastic, lipomatous, metritic, puerperal, rheumatic, scarlatinal, syphilitic, tuberculous, urethral, etc. [EU]

Syphilis: A contagious venereal disease caused by the spirochete treponema pallidum. [NIH]

Thalassemia: A group of hereditary hemolytic anemias in which there is decreased synthesis of one or more hemoglobin polypeptide chains. There are several genetic types with clinical pictures ranging from barely detectable hematologic abnormality to severe and fatal anemia. [NIH]

Thrombophlebitis: Inflammation of a vein associated with thrombus formation. [EU]

Tomography: The recording of internal body images at a predetermined plane by means of the tomograph; called also body section roentgenography. [EU]

Toxoplasmosis: An acute or chronic, widespread disease of animals and humans caused by the obligate intracellular protozoon Toxoplasma gondii, transmitted by oocysts containing the pathogen in the feces of cats (the definitive host), usually by contaminated soil, direct exposure to infected feces, tissue cysts in infected meat, or tachyzoites (proliferating forms) in blood. [EU]

Vancomycin: Antibacterial obtained from Streptomyces orientalis. It is a glycopeptide related to ristocetin that inhibits bacterial cell wall assembly and is toxic to kidneys and the inner ear. [NIH]

Varicella: Chicken pox. [EU]

Vascular: Pertaining to blood vessels or indicative of a copious blood supply. [EU]

Vestibular: Pertaining to or toward a vestibule. In dental anatomy, used to refer to the tooth surface directed toward the vestibule of the mouth. [EU]

Xerostomia: Dryness of the mouth from salivary gland dysfunction, as in Sjögren's syndrome. [EU]

CHAPTER 7. MULTIMEDIA ON SARCOIDOSIS

Overview

Information on sarcoidosis can come in a variety of formats. Among multimedia sources, video productions, slides, audiotapes, and computer databases are often available. In this chapter, we show you how to keep current on multimedia sources of information on sarcoidosis. We start with sources that have been summarized by federal agencies, and then show you how to find bibliographic information catalogued by the National Library of Medicine. If you see an interesting item, visit your local medical library to check on the availability of the title.

Video Recordings

Most diseases do not have a video dedicated to them. If they do, they are often rather technical in nature. An excellent source of multimedia information on sarcoidosis is the Combined Health Information Database. You will need to limit your search to "video recording" and "sarcoidosis" using the "Detailed Search" option. Go directly to the following hyperlink: **http://chid.nih.gov/detail/detail.html**. To find video productions, use the drop boxes at the bottom of the search page where "You may refine your search by." Select the dates and language you prefer, and the format option "Videorecording (videotape, videocassette, etc.)." By making these selections and typing "sarcoidosis" (or synonyms) into the "For these words:" box, you will only receive results on video productions. The following is a typical result when searching for video recordings on sarcoidosis:

- **Health Care Professionals' Guide to Xerostomia**

Source: Jericho, NY: Sjogren's Syndrome Foundation, Inc. 1997. (videocassette).

Contact: Available from Sjogren's Syndrome Foundation, Inc. 333 North Broadway, Jericho, NY 11753. (800) 4-SJOGREN or (516) 933-6365. Fax (516) 933-6368. Price: $29.00.

Summary: This videotape program reviews xerostomia (dry mouth). The program begins with an overview of the anatomy and physiology of the salivary glands, followed by a discussion of the three functional roles of saliva: digestion (and taste facilitation), lubrication, and protection (including antimicrobial and pH mechanisms). The narrator notes that saliva is also being used more and more as a diagnostic tool to measure systemic health. The program begins with a physician narrating, then includes interviews with two middle age women who have xerostomia; the interviews focus on the impact xerostomia has on quality of life and on the difficulties of obtaining an accurate diagnosis. The program then details the three causes of xerostomia: medical therapies (including drug side effects, radiation therapy, and surgery or trauma of the salivary glands), systemic disorders (including Sjogren's syndrome, HIV, rheumatoid arthritis, systemic lupus erythematosus, scleroderma, graft versus host disease, sarcoidosis, amyloidosis, cystic fibrosis, and neural disease affecting the salivary glands), and dehydration. The program emphasizes that xerostomia is not a natural consequence of the aging process. The program then reviews the clinical signs and oral complications of xerostomia; each is illustrated with a color photograph. Other topics include problems associated with xerostomia, the need for a multidisciplinary team approach to patients with salivary gland dysfunction, diagnostic tests used, treatment options (including chewing activity, oral moisturizing agents, and oral pilocarpine hydrochloride), determining residual salivary gland function, and the behavioral and lifestyle changes that can help patients cope with xerostomia.

Bibliography: Multimedia on Sarcoidosis

The National Library of Medicine is a rich source of information on healthcare-related multimedia productions including slides, computer software, and databases. To access the multimedia database, go to the following Web site: **http://locatorplus.gov/**. Select "Search LOCATORplus." Once in the search area, simply type in sarcoidosis (or synonyms). Then, in the option box provided below the search box, select "Audiovisuals and Computer Files." From there, you can choose to sort results by publication date, author, or relevance. The following multimedia has been indexed on sarcoidosis. For more information, follow the hyperlink indicated:

- **Continuing controversies in pulmonary disease: the nature of sarcoidosis and its therapeutic implications.** Source: Letterman General Hospital, in cooperation with Warner-Chilcott Laboratories; [made by] Television Division, Brooke Army Medical; Year: 1972; Format: Videorecording; Fort Sam Houston, Tex.: Academy of Health Sciences, [1972]

- **Cutaneous lesions : signs of internal diseases.** Source: Ervin Epstein, Ervin Epstein, Jr; Year: 1972; Format: Slide; New York: Medcom, c1972

- **Cutaneous manifestations of systemic disease.** Source: American Academy of Dermatology, and Institute for Dermatologic Communication and Education; Year: 1973; Format: Slide; [Evanston, Ill.]: The Academy, [1973]

- **Granulamatous inflammation.** Source: University of Missouri, Columbia, Medical Center, Educational Resources Group; Year: 1970; Format: Slide; Columbia: The Group, 1970

- **Granulomatous diseases of the lung.** Source: American College of Radiology Audio-visual Committee on Continuing Education; produced by 3M Company; Year: 1976; Format: Videorecording; [Chicago]: The College, c1976

- **Many faces of sarcoidosis.** Source: presented by Department of Medicine, Emory University, School of Medicine; Year: 1980; Format: Videorecording; Atlanta: Emory Medical Television Network, 1980

- **Oral manifestations of dermal lesions.** Source: produced by the American Dental Association, Council on Dental Therapeutics; Year: 1968; Format: Slide; Chicago, Ill.: The Association, 1968

- **Pulmonary disease.** Source: Whitney W. Addington; Year: 1977; Format: Sound recording; [Park Ridge, Ill.]: ASCME, p1977

- **Sarcoidosis.** Source: produced by Biomedical Communications, Univ. of Arizona Health Sciences Cntr.; presented by the American Thoracic Society, American Lung Association, ALA/ATS Committee on Learning Resources; Year: 1989; Format: Slide; [New York, N.Y.]: American Lung Association for American Thoracic Society, c1989

- **Sarcoidosis.** Source: Trainex Corporation; Year: 1975; Format: Videorecording; Garden Grove, Calif.: Trainex, c1975

- **Sarcoidosis.** Source: McMaster University, Health Sciences; Year: 1973; Format: Slide; [Hamilton, Ont.]: The University, c1973

- **Sarcoidosis.** Source: Trainex Corporation; Year: 1975; Format: Filmstrip; Garden Grove, Calif.: Trainex, p1975

Vocabulary Builder

Antimicrobial: Killing microorganisms, or suppressing their multiplication or growth. [EU]

Dehydration: The condition that results from excessive loss of body water. Called also anhydration, deaquation and hypohydration. [EU]

Digestion: The process of breakdown of food for metabolism and use by the body. [NIH]

Lubrication: The application of a substance to diminish friction between two surfaces. It may refer to oils, greases, and similar substances for the lubrication of medical equipment but it can be used for the application of substances to tissue to reduce friction, such as lotions for skin and vaginal lubricants. [NIH]

Pilocarpine: A slowly hydrolyzed muscarinic agonist with no nicotinic effects. Pilocarpine is used as a miotic and in the treatment of glaucoma. [NIH]

CHAPTER 8. PERIODICALS AND NEWS ON SARCOIDOSIS

Overview

Keeping up on the news relating to sarcoidosis can be challenging. Subscribing to targeted periodicals can be an effective way to stay abreast of recent developments on sarcoidosis. Periodicals include newsletters, magazines, and academic journals.

In this chapter, we suggest a number of news sources and present various periodicals that cover sarcoidosis beyond and including those which are published by patient associations mentioned earlier. We will first focus on news services, and then on periodicals. News services, press releases, and newsletters generally use more accessible language, so if you do chose to subscribe to one of the more technical periodicals, make sure that it uses language you can easily follow.

News Services & Press Releases

Well before articles show up in newsletters or the popular press, they may appear in the form of a press release or a public relations announcement. One of the simplest ways of tracking press releases on sarcoidosis is to search the news wires. News wires are used by professional journalists, and have existed since the invention of the telegraph. Today, there are several major "wires" that are used by companies, universities, and other organizations to announce new medical breakthroughs. In the following sample of sources, we will briefly describe how to access each service. These services only post recent news intended for public viewing.

PR Newswire

Perhaps the broadest of the wires is PR Newswire Association, Inc. To access this archive, simply go to **http://www.prnewswire.com**. Below the search box, select the option "The last 30 days." In the search box, type "sarcoidosis" or synonyms. The search results are shown by order of relevance. When reading these press releases, do not forget that the sponsor of the release may be a company or organization that is trying to sell a particular product or therapy. Their views, therefore, may be biased.

Reuters

The Reuters' Medical News database can be very useful in exploring news archives relating to sarcoidosis. While some of the listed articles are free to view, others can be purchased for a nominal fee. To access this archive, go to **http://www.reutershealth.com/frame2/arch.html** and search by "sarcoidosis" (or synonyms). The following was recently listed in this archive for sarcoidosis:

- **Instance reported of IL-2 therapy triggering HAART-induced sarcoidosis**
  Source: Reuters Medical News
  Date: January 10, 2001
  http://www.reuters.gov/archive/2001/01/10/professional/links/20010110clin007.html

- **Sputum useful to investigate inflammation markers in sarcoidosis patients**
  Source: Reuters Medical News
  Date: August 18, 2000
  http://www.reuters.gov/archive/2000/08/18/professional/links/20000818clin004.html

- **Sarcoidosis may be a risk factor for variety of cancers**
  Source: Reuters Medical News
  Date: November 23, 1999
  http://www.reuters.gov/archive/1999/11/23/professional/links/19991123epid003.html

- **Sarcoidosis on Aircraft Carriers**
  Source: Reuters Health eLine
  Date: June 16, 1997
  http://www.reuters.gov/archive/1997/06/16/eline/links/19970616elin008.html

- **Corticosteroids Linked To Increased Risk Of Relapse In Sarcoidosis**
Source: Reuters Medical News
Date: March 28, 1997
http://www.reuters.gov/archive/1997/03/28/professional/links/19970328clin004.html

The NIH

Within MEDLINEplus, the NIH has made an agreement with the New York Times Syndicate, the AP News Service, and Reuters to deliver news that can be browsed by the public. Search news releases at **http://www.nlm.nih.gov/medlineplus/alphanews_a.html.** MEDLINEplus allows you to browse across an alphabetical index. Or you can search by date at **http://www.nlm.nih.gov/medlineplus/newsbydate.html**. Often, news items are indexed by MEDLINEplus within their search engine.

Business Wire

Business Wire is similar to PR Newswire. To access this archive, simply go to **http://www.businesswire.com**. You can scan the news by industry category or company name.

Internet Wire

Internet Wire is more focused on technology than the other wires. To access this site, go to **http://www.internetwire.com** and use the "Search Archive" option. Type in "sarcoidosis" (or synonyms). As this service is oriented to technology, you may wish to search for press releases covering diagnostic procedures or tests that you may have read about.

Search Engines

Free-to-view news can also be found in the news section of your favorite search engines (see the health news page at Yahoo: **http://dir.yahoo.com/Health/News_and_Media/,** or use this Web site's general news search page **http://news.yahoo.com/.** Type in "sarcoidosis" (or synonyms). If you know the name of a company that is relevant to sarcoidosis, you can go to any stock trading Web site (such as **www.etrade.com**) and search for the company name there. News items across various news sources are reported on indicated hyperlinks.

BBC

Covering news from a more European perspective, the British Broadcasting Corporation (BBC) allows the public free access to their news archive located at **http://www.bbc.co.uk/**. Search by "sarcoidosis" (or synonyms).

Newsletters on Sarcoidosis

Given their focus on current and relevant developments, newsletters are often more useful to patients than academic articles. You can find newsletters using the Combined Health Information Database (CHID). You will need to use the "Detailed Search" option. To access CHID, go directly to the following hyperlink: **http://chid.nih.gov/detail/detail.html**. Your investigation must limit the search to "Newsletter" and "sarcoidosis." Go to the bottom of the search page where "You may refine your search by." Select the dates and language that you prefer. For the format option, select "Newsletter." By making these selections and typing in "sarcoidosis" or synonyms into the "For these words:" box, you will only receive results on newsletters. The following list was generated using the options described above:

- **Kidney Failure in Sarcoidosis**

  Source: Sarcoidosis Networking. 8(3): 3. 2000.

  Contact: Available from Sarcoid Network Association. Sarcoidosis Networking, 13925 80th Street East, Puyallup, WA 98372-3614. Email: sarcoidosis_network@prodigy.net.

  Summary: Sarcoidosis is a chronic, progressive systemic granulomatous (causing lesions) disease of unknown cause (etiology), involving almost any organ or tissue, including the skin, lungs, lymph nodes, liver, spleen, eyes, and small bones of the hands or feet. This brief article, from a newsletter for patients with sarcoidosis, reviews the complications of kidney failure in sarcoidosis. Granulomatous infiltration of the kidney may be present in as many as 40 percent of patients with sarcoidosis, but it is rarely extensive enough to cause renal (kidney) dysfunction. The lesions are usually responsive to steroid therapy. Kidney failure has also been diagnosed in patients with sarcoidosis without the presence of lesions, possibly due to hypercalcemia (too much calcium in the blood), involvement of the glomerular filter system, and renal arteritis (inflammation of the arteries of the kidney), which may be associated with severe high blood pressure. It is recommended that all people with active sarcoidosis be screened for hypercalciuria (high levels of calcium in the urine). This may precede development of hypercalcemia, which should be treated. Glucocorticoids are the main choice of therapy and do seem to reduce levels of urinary calcium to normal within a few days. People with sarcoidosis may also have severe pain; the frequent use of pain medication can be another cause of kidney failure. People who take pain medication should ask their physicians to evaluate their kidneys on a regular basis. 9 references.

- **Kidney Disease**

Source: Sarcoidosis Networking. 8(3): 2. May-June 2000.

Contact: Available from Sarcoid Network Association. Sarcoidosis Networking, 13925 80th Street East, Puyallup, WA 98372-3614. Email: sarcoidosis_network@prodigy.net.

Summary: Sarcoidosis is a chronic, progressive systemic granulomatous (causing lesions) disease of unknown cause (etiology), involving almost any organ or tissue, including the skin, lungs, lymph nodes, liver, spleen, eyes, and small bones of the hands or feet. This brief article, from a newsletter for patients with sarcoidosis, reviews kidney disease, its types, diagnosis, and management. The article begins with a summary of the anatomy and function of the kidneys, which filter the blood (removing waste and excess body fluids), and maintain the balance of some essential nutrients helping to regulate blood pressure, red blood cells, and elements such as potassium and calcium. Without functioning kidneys, one cannot live without dialysis, the mechanical filtration of the blood. Kidneys fail for a variety of reasons, including trauma to the kidney, toxins, heart failure, obstruction (kidney stones), overuse of some medications, and diseases that invade the kidney, such as sarcoidosis. Diabetes and high blood pressure are the most common causes for loss of kidney function. Warning signs of kidney disease are high blood pressure (hypertension), blood or protein in the urine, creatinine level greater than 1.2 in women or 1.4 in men, more frequent urination (especially at night), difficult or painful urination, and puffy eyes or swelling of the hands or feet (especially in children). Loss of kidney function can produce symptoms including fatigue, weakness, nausea, vomiting, diarrhea or constipation, headaches, loss of appetite, increased edema (fluid retention), and fever or chills. Kidney failure is characterized as acute kidney failure, chronic kidney insufficiency, and chronic kidney failure. The need to put a person on dialysis depends upon the levels of creatinine and urea nitrogen in the blood and the evaluation of body parameters such as fluid status, and symptoms of toxicity. The author encourages readers to practice preventive measures which include drinking 8 to 10 glasses of water per day, preventing or treating diabetes and high blood pressure, avoiding tobacco, eating a well balanced diet, practicing good hygiene, treating wounds and infections, limiting exposure to heavy metals and toxic chemicals, and avoiding unnecessary over the counter drug use.

Newsletter Articles

If you choose not to subscribe to a newsletter, you can nevertheless find references to newsletter articles. We recommend that you use the Combined Health Information Database, while limiting your search criteria to "newsletter articles." Again, you will need to use the "Detailed Search" option. To search the Combined Health Information Database go directly to the following hyperlink: **http://chid.nih.gov/detail/detail.html**. Go to the bottom of the search page where "You may refine your search by." Select the dates and language that you prefer. For the format option, select "Newsletter Article."

By making these selections, and typing in "sarcoidosis" (or synonyms) into the "For these words:" box, you will only receive results on newsletter articles. You should check back periodically with this database as it is updated every 3 months. The following is a typical result when searching for newsletter articles on sarcoidosis:

- **Dry Eyes**

   Source: EDucator, The. p. 3-4. November-December 2000.

   Contact: Available from National Foundation for Ectodermal Dysplasias. 410 East Main Street, P.O. Box 114, Mascoutah, IL 62258-0114. (618) 566-2020. Fax (618) 566-4718. Website: www.nfed.org.

   Summary: This newsletter article provides people who have dry eyes with information on the causes, categories, and treatment of this condition. Various environmental influences, medical disorders, and medications may cause dry eyes, which can be divided into two major groups: those in which there is inadequate production of the watery component of tears and those in which there is adequate watery tear production. Inadequate production of the watery component of tears results from an undersecreting tear gland. Conditions associated with tear deficiency include congenital alacrima, lymphoma, sarcoidosis, amyloidosis, severe vitamin A deficiency, neurologic conditions, and Sjogren's syndrome. One cause of dry eyes with adequate watery tear production is abnormal functioning of the oil glands in the eyelids that produce the protective oily layer on the outside of the tear film. Other conditions that increase tear film evaporation include increased width of the eyelids and inadequate lid closure. The treatment of irritation with dry eyes is mainly directed at symptom relief. The usual treatment for decreased aqueous tear production is topically applied lubricants and ointments. Other treatment options include humidifying the indoor environment, placing side panels and moisture chambers around the frame of eyeglasses, covering the eyes at night to reduce tear evaporation, and occluding the punctum with small collagen plugs.

- **Use of Methotrexate in Children**

Source: Bulletin on the Rheumatic Diseases. 47(5): 1-5. August 1998.

Contact: Available from Arthritis Foundation. 1330 West Peachtree Street, Atlanta, GA 30309. (404) 872-7100. Fax (404) 872-9559.

Summary: This newsletter article provides health professionals with information on the use of methotrexate to treat rheumatic diseases in children. A double blind, placebo controlled study found that low dose methotrexate was the only second line drug to be effective in the treatment of juvenile rheumatoid arthritis (JRA). However, there are no predictors to indicate whether an individual patient will respond to methotrexate therapy. In addition, it is unclear whether methotrexate can modify the course of JRA and how long to continue methotrexate after remission is achieved. Methotrexate also shows promise in treating inflammatory ocular disease, juvenile dermatomyositis, sarcoidosis, inflammatory bowel disease, and vasculitic syndromes. Methotrexate is generally well tolerated in children, and side effects are usually mild and transient. Most commonly noted are gastrointestinal side effects on the day methotrexate is taken. Oral mucosal ulcerations also occur frequently. Most patients usually have transient liver biochemical abnormalities at least once during methotrexate therapy. Hematologic, infectious, and pulmonary toxicities are rarely seen in children. Methotrexate is highly teratogenic, so counseling and management strategies should be used with adolescent girls who may be or may become sexually active. Adolescent patients taking methotrexate must also be cautioned against the use of alcohol. Varicella vaccine should be given to unexposed patients at least 3 weeks before initiating methotrexate therapy. Methotrexate therapy should be discontinued in patients who develop Epstein-Barr virus infection. Various laboratory tests should be obtained at baseline, 2 weeks, and every 4 to 8 weeks thereafter. The role of the primary care physician in the management of a disease treated with methotrexate is to treat interim infection and alert the specialist if discontinuation of methotrexate is warranted. 2 tables and 23 references.

- **Safe Fun in the Sun**

  Source: Sarcoidosis Networking. 4; May/June 1997.

  Contact: Sarcoid Networking Association, 13925 80th Street East, Puyallup, WA 98372-3614. (253) 845-3108. (253) 845-3108 (fax).

  Summary: This newsletter article for individuals with sarcoidosis offers guidelines for avoiding the health dangers of the sun. Suggestions include planning outdoor activities for early morning or late afternoon, using a broad-spectrum ultraviolet (UV) A and B sunscreen, reapplying sunscreen when swimming or perspiring, wearing sunglasses that screen out both UVA and UVB, and examining the skin for unusual moles or other skin features.

- **You Asked**

  Source: Sarcoidosis Networking. 10; September/October 1997.

  Contact: Pacific Northwest Sarcoid Association, Sarcoid Networking Association, 13925 80th Street East, Puyallup, WA 98372-3614. (253) 845-3108. (253) 845-3108 (fax).

  Summary: This newsletter article for individuals with sarcoidosis answers questions about this disease. Questions address the issues of whether sarcoidosis and its associated skin rash are contagious; whether this disease is a form of cancer, acquired immune deficiency syndrome, or Hodgkin's Disease; and whether it is an allergic disease or can develop into asthma. Other questions deal with features that indicate whether sarcoidosis is serious, whether sarcoidosis causes diabetes, and whether shortness of breath could be fatal in an asthma attack.

- **Sarcoidosis**

  Source: Sarcoidosis Networking. 2-3; September/October 1997.

  Contact: Pacific Northwest Sarcoid Association, Sarcoid Networking Association, 13925 80th Street East, Puyallup, WA 98372-3614. (253) 845-3108. (253) 845-3108 (fax).

  Summary: This newsletter article for individuals with sarcoidosis presents an overview of this disease. Sarcoidosis spreads white blood cells throughout the body, and they clump together and form a mass known as granuloma. A granuloma that grows large enough may then block the function of any body tissue. The article describes the symptoms of sarcoidosis, presents the techniques used to diagnosis sarcoidosis, identifies the drugs used to treat the symptoms of sarcoidosis, and highlights the side effects of these drugs. 16 references.

- **Back First Aid**

  Source: Sarcoidosis Networking. 3; September/October 1997.

  Contact: Pacific Northwest Sarcoid Association, Sarcoid Networking Association, 13925 80th Street East, Puyallup, WA 98372-3614. (253) 845-3108. (253) 845-3108 (fax).

  Summary: This newsletter article for individuals with sarcoidosis presents Agency for Health Care Policy and Research (AHCPR) recommendations for managing active low back pain. Recommendations include halting the activity triggering the pain, modifying other activities, controlling the pain by taking acetaminophen or nonsteroidal anti-inflammatory drugs, and considering consulting a chiropractor or osteopath for a short course of manipulation. The AHCPR found inconclusive evidence to recommend various alternative therapies. 1 reference.

- **Getting Shoes That Fit**

  Source: Sarcoidosis Networking. 5(6):3; November/December 1997.

  Contact: Pacific Northwest Sarcoid Association, Sarcoid Networking Association, 13925 80th Street East, Puyallup, WA 98372-3614. (253) 845-3108. (253) 845-3108 (fax).

  Summary: This newsletter article for individuals with sarcoidosis presents guidelines for purchasing shoes that are comfortable and are a good fit. Suggestions for finding a pair of comfortable, well-fitting shoes include walking without shoes several times back and forth in front of a full length mirror to observe gait, arm swing, and hip movement; repeating this process with one's present shoes; shopping for shoes half way through the day; observing gait, arm swing, and hip movement in a potential new pair of shoes; walking around the house in the new pair of shoes and observing gait, arm swing, and hip movement in a full length mirror; and examining one's feet for any signs of irritation from the new shoes.

- **Rapidly Progressive Sensorineural Hearing Loss**

  Source: Sarcoidosis Networking. 8(3): 9. May-June 2000.

  Contact: Available from Sarcoidosis Networking Association. 13925 80th Street East, Puyallup, WA 98372-3614. E-mail: sarcoidosis_networking@prodigy.net.

Summary: This brief article, from a newsletter for people with sarcoidosis, describes rapidly progressive sensorineural hearing loss (SNHL). The author first defines three types of hearing loss: conductive, sensorineural, and mixed. The author then notes that sudden SNHL is of great concern and may be caused by various factors. Every patient with SNHL should be evaluated thoroughly to determine the underlying disorder contributing to the hearing loss. Early diagnosis of SNHL is crucial as a significant number of patients with idiopathic (unknown cause) SNHL may have an immunological condition causing their hearing loss. The author reviews the diagnostic tests commonly used to evaluate idiopathic progressive SNHL and stresses the importance of prompt and effective treatment. Patients with autoimmune deafness may benefit from immunosuppressive therapy.

- **Skin Sarcoidosis**

Source: Sarcoidosis Networking. 7(4): 2. July-August 1999.

Contact: Available from Sarcoidosis Networking. 13925 80th Street East, Puyallup, WA 98372-3614. (253) 845-3108. E-mail: VBKR29A@prodigy.com.

Summary: This newsletter article provides people who have sarcoidosis with information on the skin lesions associated with this multisystem granulomatous disease of unknown cause. Skin lesions of sarcoidosis are classified as specific and nonspecific. Biopsy of lesions of the specific type show evidence of granulomas, whereas no granuloma tissue is found in the biopsy for the nonspecific type. Erythema nodosum is an example of this latter form. Papule lesions are the most common and usually have a brownish or reddish brown hue. The sarcoid lesions of lupus pernio, which are reddish, purple leash clusters, are more common among African Americans than Caucasians. Sarcoid granulomas found in scar tissue form bumps or nodules, making the scar appear reddish or purple. These are often called keloid formations. A very invasive form of sarcoidosis is a loss of hair where granulomas infiltrate and destroy the hair follicles. Ulcerative sarcoid lesions are mainly seen on lower extremities. Dairier-Roussy lesions are asymptomatic, subcutaneous lesions that can appear over the trunk and extremities under the surface skin. Psoriasiform changes, which are rare, look like psoriasis on the trunk and extremities. Treatment options include topical or systemic corticosteroids. Good personal hygiene is very important in preventing skin breakdown.

Academic Periodicals covering Sarcoidosis

Academic periodicals can be a highly technical yet valuable source of information on sarcoidosis. We have compiled the following list of periodicals known to publish articles relating to sarcoidosis and which are currently indexed within the National Library of Medicine's PubMed database (follow hyperlinks to view more information, summaries, etc., for each). In addition to these sources, to keep current on articles written on sarcoidosis published by any of the periodicals listed below, you can simply follow the hyperlink indicated or go to the following Web site: **www.ncbi.nlm.nih.gov/pubmed**. Type the periodical's name into the search box to find the latest studies published.

If you want complete details about the historical contents of a periodical, you can also visit **http://www.ncbi.nlm.nih.gov/entrez/jrbrowser.cgi**. Here, type in the name of the journal or its abbreviation, and you will receive an index of published articles. At **http://locatorplus.gov/** you can retrieve more indexing information on medical periodicals (e.g. the name of the publisher). Select the button "Search LOCATORplus." Then type in the name of the journal and select the advanced search option "Journal Title Search." The following is a sample of periodicals which publish articles on sarcoidosis:

- **Annals of Hematology. (Ann Hematol)**
  http://www.ncbi.nlm.nih.gov/entrez/jrbrowser.cgi?field=0&regexp=Annals+of+Hematology&dispmax=20&dispstart=0

- **Annals of Internal Medicine. (Ann Intern Med)**
  http://www.ncbi.nlm.nih.gov/entrez/jrbrowser.cgi?field=0&regexp=Annals+of+Internal+Medicine&dispmax=20&dispstart=0

- **Archives of Internal Medicine. (Arch Intern Med)**
  http://www.ncbi.nlm.nih.gov/entrez/jrbrowser.cgi?field=0&regexp=Archives+of+Internal+Medicine&dispmax=20&dispstart=0

- **Bmj (Clinical Research Ed. . (BMJ)**
  http://www.ncbi.nlm.nih.gov/entrez/jrbrowser.cgi?field=0&regexp=Bmj+(Clinical+Research+Ed.+&dispmax=20&dispstart=0

- **Clinical and Experimental Immunology. (Clin Exp Immunol)**
  http://www.ncbi.nlm.nih.gov/entrez/jrbrowser.cgi?field=0&regexp=Cli
  nical+and+Experimental+Immunology&dispmax=20&dispstart=0

- **Journal of Internal Medicine. (J Intern Med)**
  http://www.ncbi.nlm.nih.gov/entrez/jrbrowser.cgi?field=0&regexp=Jo
  urnal+of+Internal+Medicine&dispmax=20&dispstart=0

- **Leukemia & Lymphoma. (Leuk Lymphoma)**
  http://www.ncbi.nlm.nih.gov/entrez/jrbrowser.cgi?field=0&regexp=Le
  ukemia+&+Lymphoma&dispmax=20&dispstart=0

- **Medical and Pediatric Oncology. (Med Pediatr Oncol)**
  http://www.ncbi.nlm.nih.gov/entrez/jrbrowser.cgi?field=0&regexp=M
  edical+and+Pediatric+Oncology&dispmax=20&dispstart=0

- **Proceedings of the National Academy of Sciences of the United States
  of America. (Proc Natl Acad Sci U S A)**
  http://www.ncbi.nlm.nih.gov/entrez/jrbrowser.cgi?field=0&regexp=Pr
  oceedings+of+the+National+Academy+of+Sciences+of+the+United+Stat
  es+of+America&dispmax=20&dispstart=0

- **Respiratory Medicine. (Respir Med)**
  http://www.ncbi.nlm.nih.gov/entrez/jrbrowser.cgi?field=0&regexp=Re
  spiratory+Medicine&dispmax=20&dispstart=0

- **The American Journal of Medicine. (Am J Med)**
  http://www.ncbi.nlm.nih.gov/entrez/jrbrowser.cgi?field=0&regexp=Th
  e+American+Journal+of+Medicine&dispmax=20&dispstart=0

- **The British Journal of Dermatology. (Br J Dermatol)**
  http://www.ncbi.nlm.nih.gov/entrez/jrbrowser.cgi?field=0&regexp=Th
  e+British+Journal+of+Dermatology&dispmax=20&dispstart=0

- **The Journal of Clinical Investigation. (J Clin Invest)**
  http://www.ncbi.nlm.nih.gov/entrez/jrbrowser.cgi?field=0&regexp=Th
  e+Journal+of+Clinical+Investigation&dispmax=20&dispstart=0

- **The Journal of Laboratory and Clinical Medicine. (J Lab Clin Med)**
  http://www.ncbi.nlm.nih.gov/entrez/jrbrowser.cgi?field=0&regexp=The+Journal+of+Laboratory+and+Clinical+Medicine&dispmax=20&dispstart=0

Vocabulary Builder

Acetaminophen: Analgesic antipyretic derivative of acetanilide. It has weak anti-inflammatory properties and is used as a common analgesic, but may cause liver, blood cell, and kidney damage. [NIH]

Arteries: The vessels carrying blood away from the heart. [NIH]

Constipation: Infrequent or difficult evacuation of the faeces. [EU]

Diarrhea: Passage of excessively liquid or excessively frequent stools. [NIH]

Invasive: 1. having the quality of invasiveness. 2. involving puncture or incision of the skin or insertion of an instrument or foreign material into the body; said of diagnostic techniques. [EU]

Keloid: A sharply elevated, irregularly- shaped, progressively enlarging scar due to the formation of excessive amounts of collagen in the corium during connective tissue repair. [EU]

Nausea: An unpleasant sensation, vaguely referred to the epigastrium and abdomen, and often culminating in vomiting. [EU]

Ointments: Semisolid preparations used topically for protective emollient effects or as a vehicle for local administration of medications. Ointment bases are various mixtures of fats, waxes, animal and plant oils and solid and liquid hydrocarbons. [NIH]

Papule: A small circumscribed, superficial, solid elevation of the skin. [EU]

Psoriasis: A common genetically determined, chronic, inflammatory skin disease characterized by rounded erythematous, dry, scaling patches. The lesions have a predilection for nails, scalp, genitalia, extensor surfaces, and the lumbosacral region. Accelerated epidermopoiesis is considered to be the fundamental pathologic feature in psoriasis. [NIH]

Teratogenic: Tending to produce anomalies of formation, or teratism (= anomaly of formation or development : condition of a monster). [EU]

Toxin: A poison; frequently used to refer specifically to a protein produced by some higher plants, certain animals, and pathogenic bacteria, which is highly toxic for other living organisms. Such substances are differentiated from the simple chemical poisons and the vegetable alkaloids by their high molecular weight and antigenicity. [EU]

Vaccine: A suspension of attenuated or killed microorganisms (bacteria, viruses, or rickettsiae), administered for the prevention, amelioration or treatment of infectious diseases. [EU]

CHAPTER 9. PHYSICIAN GUIDELINES AND DATABASES

Overview

Doctors and medical researchers rely on a number of information sources to help patients with their conditions. Many will subscribe to journals or newsletters published by their professional associations or refer to specialized textbooks or clinical guides published for the medical profession. In this chapter, we focus on databases and Internet-based guidelines created or written for this professional audience.

NIH Guidelines

For the more common diseases, The National Institutes of Health publish guidelines that are frequently consulted by physicians. Publications are typically written by one or more of the various NIH Institutes. For physician guidelines, commonly referred to as "clinical" or "professional" guidelines, you can visit the following Institutes:

- Office of the Director (OD); guidelines consolidated across agencies available at **http://www.nih.gov/health/consumer/conkey.htm**

- National Institute of General Medical Sciences (NIGMS); fact sheets available at **http://www.nigms.nih.gov/news/facts/**

- National Library of Medicine (NLM); extensive encyclopedia (A.D.A.M., Inc.) with guidelines:
  http://www.nlm.nih.gov/medlineplus/healthtopics.html

- National Heart, Lung, and Blood Institute (NHLBI); guidelines available at **http://www.nhlbi.nih.gov/guidelines/index.htm**

The NHLBI recently recommended the following guidelines and references to physicians treating patients with lung conditions:

Asthma

General:

- National Asthma Education and Prevention Program Slide Sets: **http://hin.nhlbi.nih.gov/naepp_slds/menu.htm**

- Action Against Asthma: A Strategic Plan for the Department of Health and Human Services: **http://aspe.hhs.gov/sp/asthma**

- Asthma Management Model System (Web Site): **http://www.nhlbisupport.com/asthma/index.html**

- Asthma Management in Minority Children: **http://www.nhlbi.nih.gov/health/prof/lung/asthma/ast_chil.htm**

- AsthmaMemo: **http://www.nhlbi.nih.gov/health/prof/lung/asthma/asth_mem.htm**

- Data Fact Sheet: Asthma Statistics: **http://www.nhlbi.nih.gov/health/prof/lung/asthma/asthstat.htm**

- Diagnosing and Managing Asthma in the Elderly: **http://www.nhlbi.nih.gov/health/prof/lung/asthma/as_elder.htm**

- Guidelines for the Diagnosis and Management of Asthma: NAEPP Expert Panel Report 2: **http://www.nhlbi.nih.gov/guidelines/asthma/asthgdln.htm**

- NAEPP Task Force on the Cost Effectiveness, Quality of Care, and Financing of Asthma Care: **http://www.nhlbi.nih.gov/health/prof/lung/asthma/ast_cost.htm**

- Nurses: Partners in Asthma Care: **http://www.nhlbi.nih.gov/health/prof/lung/asthma/nurs_gde.htm**

- Practical Guide for the Diagnosis and Management of Asthma: **http://www.nhlbi.nih.gov/health/prof/lung/asthma/practgde.htm**

- Report of the Working Group on Asthma and Pregnancy: **http://www.nhlbi.nih.gov/health/prof/lung/asthma/astpreg.txt**

- The Role of the Pharmacist in Improving Asthma Care: **http://www.nhlbi.nih.gov/health/prof/lung/asthma/asmapmcy.htm**

- World Asthma Day 2001 (May 3, 2001): **http://www.nhlbi.nih.gov/health/prof/lung/asthma/wad_2/index.htm**

Schools/child care centers:

- NAEPP Resolution on Asthma Management at School:
  http://www.nhlbi.nih.gov/health/public/lung/asthma/resolut.htm

- Asthma and Physical Activity in the School:
  http://www.nhlbi.nih.gov/health/public/lung/asthma/phy_asth.htm

- Asthma Awareness Curriculum for the Elementary Classroom:
  http://www.nhlbi.nih.gov/health/prof/lung/asthma/school/index.htm

- How Asthma-Friendly Is Your School? (¿Su escuela tiene en cuenta a los niños con asma?):
  http://www.nhlbi.nih.gov/health/public/lung/asthma/friendhi.htm

- How Asthma-Friendly Is Your Child-Care Setting? (¿Su guardería infantil tiene en cuenta a los niños con asma?):
  http://www.nhlbi.nih.gov/health/public/lung/asthma/child_ca.htm

- School Asthma Education Slide Set:
  http://hin.nhlbi.nih.gov/naepp_slds/menu.htm

See also:

- Asthma Clinical Research Network (ACRN): **http://www.acrn.org/**[28]

- Global Initiative for Asthma:
  http://www.nhlbi.nih.gov/health/prof/lung/gina.htm

- National Asthma Education and Prevention Program:
  http://www.nhlbi.nih.gov/about/naepp/index.htm

National Emphysema Treatment Trial (NETT)

- News Release: NHLBI-Funded Emphysema Study Finds Certain Patients at High Risk for Death Following Lung Surgery, August 14, 2001:
  http://www.nhlbi.nih.gov/new/press/01-08-14.htm

- News Release: NHLBI/HCFA Lung Volume Reduction Surgery Study Participants Announced, December 20, 1996:
  http://www.nhlbi.nih.gov/health/prof/lung/nett/lvrspr.htm

- Background and Study Information:
  http://www.nhlbi.nih.gov/health/prof/lung/nett/lvrsweb.htm

---

[28] Please note: This link, which goes outside the NHLBI Web site, will open a new browser window; to return to this document, either close the new window, or toggle back (ALT-TAB for Windows users, Apple-TAB for Macintosh users).

- Participating Centers:
  http://www.nhlbi.nih.gov/health/prof/lung/nett/lvrsctr.htm

Other Pulmonary Information

Global Initiative for Chronic Obstructive Lung Disease (GOLD):

- COPD Guideline Tool for Palm OS: http://hin.nhlbi.nih.gov/copd.htm

- Workshop Report: http://www.nhlbi.nih.gov/health/prof/lung/gold.htm

- Tuberculosis Academic Awards:
  http://www.nhlbi.nih.gov/funding/training/tbaa/index.htm

- Acute Respiratory Distress Syndrome Clinical Network (ARDSNet):
  http://hedwig.mgh.harvard.edu/ardsnet/

- Pulmonary Immunobiology and Inflammation in Pulmonary Diseases
  NHLBI, Workshop Summary:
  http://www.nhlbi.nih.gov/meetings/workshops/pul_inflam.htm

- Pharmacological Therapy for Idiopathic Pulmonary Fibrosis: Past,
  Present, and Future, NHLBI Workshop Summary:
  http://www.nhlbi.nih.gov/meetings/workshops/ipf-sum.htm

- Nurses: Help Your Patients Stop Smoking:
  http://www.nhlbi.nih.gov/health/prof/lung/other/nurssmok.txt

See also:

- List of Publications:
  http://www.nhlbi.nih.gov/health/pubs/pub_prof.htm

- Information Center: http://www.nhlbi.nih.gov/health/infoctr/index.htm

- Lung Information for Patients/Public:
  http://www.nhlbi.nih.gov/health/public/lung/index.htm

NIH Databases

In addition to the various Institutes of Health that publish professional
guidelines, the NIH has designed a number of databases for professionals.[29]

---

[29] Remember, for the general public, the National Library of Medicine recommends the
databases referenced in MEDLINE*plus* (http://medlineplus.gov/ or
http://www.nlm.nih.gov/medlineplus/databases.html).

Physician-oriented resources provide a wide variety of information related to the biomedical and health sciences, both past and present. The format of these resources varies. Searchable databases, bibliographic citations, full text articles (when available), archival collections, and images are all available. The following are referenced by the National Library of Medicine:[30]

- **Bioethics:** Access to published literature on the ethical, legal and public policy issues surrounding healthcare and biomedical research. This information is provided in conjunction with the Kennedy Institute of Ethics located at Georgetown University, Washington, D.C.: **http://www.nlm.nih.gov/databases/databases_bioethics.html**

- **HIV/AIDS Resources:** Describes various links and databases dedicated to HIV/AIDS research: **http://www.nlm.nih.gov/pubs/factsheets/aidsinfs.html**

- **NLM Online Exhibitions:** Describes "Exhibitions in the History of Medicine": **http://www.nlm.nih.gov/exhibition/exhibition.html**. Additional resources for historical scholarship in medicine: **http://www.nlm.nih.gov/hmd/hmd.html**

- **Biotechnology Information:** Access to public databases. The National Center for Biotechnology Information conducts research in computational biology, develops software tools for analyzing genome data, and disseminates biomedical information for the better understanding of molecular processes affecting human health and disease: **http://www.ncbi.nlm.nih.gov/**

- **Population Information:** The National Library of Medicine provides access to worldwide coverage of population, family planning, and related health issues, including family planning technology and programs, fertility, and population law and policy: **http://www.nlm.nih.gov/databases/databases_population.html**

- **Cancer Information:** Access to caner-oriented databases: **http://www.nlm.nih.gov/databases/databases_cancer.html**

- **Profiles in Science:** Offering the archival collections of prominent twentieth-century biomedical scientists to the public through modern digital technology: **http://www.profiles.nlm.nih.gov/**

- **Chemical Information:** Provides links to various chemical databases and references: **http://sis.nlm.nih.gov/Chem/ChemMain.html**

- **Clinical Alerts:** Reports the release of findings from the NIH-funded clinical trials where such release could significantly affect morbidity and mortality: **http://www.nlm.nih.gov/databases/alerts/clinical_alerts.html**

---

[30] See **http://www.nlm.nih.gov/databases/databases.html**.

- **Space Life Sciences:** Provides links and information to space-based research (including NASA):
  http://www.nlm.nih.gov/databases/databases_space.html

- **MEDLINE:** Bibliographic database covering the fields of medicine, nursing, dentistry, veterinary medicine, the healthcare system, and the pre-clinical sciences:
  http://www.nlm.nih.gov/databases/databases_medline.html

- **Toxicology and Environmental Health Information (TOXNET):** Databases covering toxicology and environmental health:
  http://sis.nlm.nih.gov/Tox/ToxMain.html

- **Visible Human Interface:** Anatomically detailed, three-dimensional representations of normal male and female human bodies:
  http://www.nlm.nih.gov/research/visible/visible_human.html

While all of the above references may be of interest to physicians who study and treat sarcoidosis, the following are particularly noteworthy.

The NLM Gateway[31]

The NLM (National Library of Medicine) Gateway is a Web-based system that lets users search simultaneously in multiple retrieval systems at the U.S. National Library of Medicine (NLM). It allows users of NLM services to initiate searches from one Web interface, providing "one-stop searching" for many of NLM's information resources or databases.[32] One target audience for the Gateway is the Internet user who is new to NLM's online resources and does not know what information is available or how best to search for it. This audience may include physicians and other healthcare providers, researchers, librarians, students, and, increasingly, patients, their families, and the public.[33] To use the NLM Gateway, simply go to the search site at

[31] Adapted from NLM: **http://gateway.nlm.nih.gov/gw/Cmd?Overview.x**.
[32] The NLM Gateway is currently being developed by the Lister Hill National Center for Biomedical Communications (LHNCBC) at the National Library of Medicine (NLM) of the National Institutes of Health (NIH).
[33] Other users may find the Gateway useful for an overall search of NLM's information resources. Some searchers may locate what they need immediately, while others will utilize the Gateway as an adjunct tool to other NLM search services such as PubMed® and MEDLINEplus®. The Gateway connects users with multiple NLM retrieval systems while also providing a search interface for its own collections. These collections include various types of information that do not logically belong in PubMed, LOCATORplus, or other established NLM retrieval systems (e.g., meeting announcements and pre-1966 journal citations). The Gateway will provide access to the information found in an increasing number of NLM retrieval systems in several phases.

http://gateway.nlm.nih.gov/gw/Cmd. Type "sarcoidosis" (or synonyms) into the search box and click "Search." The results will be presented in a tabular form, indicating the number of references in each database category.

Results Summary

Category	Items Found
Journal Articles	15976
Books / Periodicals / Audio Visual	149
Consumer Health	51
Meeting Abstracts	8
Other Collections	0
Total	16184

HSTAT[34]

HSTAT is a free, Web-based resource that provides access to full-text documents used in healthcare decision-making.[35] HSTAT's audience includes healthcare providers, health service researchers, policy makers, insurance companies, consumers, and the information professionals who serve these groups. HSTAT provides access to a wide variety of publications, including clinical practice guidelines, quick-reference guides for clinicians, consumer health brochures, evidence reports and technology assessments from the Agency for Healthcare Research and Quality (AHRQ), as well as AHRQ's Put Prevention Into Practice.[36] Simply search by "sarcoidosis" (or synonyms) at the following Web site: **http://text.nlm.nih.gov**.

---

[34] Adapted from HSTAT: **http://www.nlm.nih.gov/pubs/factsheets/hstat.html**
[35] The HSTAT URL is **http://hstat.nlm.nih.gov/**.
[36] Other important documents in HSTAT include: the National Institutes of Health (NIH) Consensus Conference Reports and Technology Assessment Reports; the HIV/AIDS Treatment Information Service (ATIS) resource documents; the Substance Abuse and Mental Health Services Administration's Center for Substance Abuse Treatment (SAMHSA/CSAT) Treatment Improvement Protocols (TIP) and Center for Substance Abuse Prevention (SAMHSA/CSAP) Prevention Enhancement Protocols System (PEPS); the Public Health Service (PHS) Preventive Services Task Force's *Guide to Clinical Preventive Services*; the independent, nonfederal Task Force on Community Services *Guide to Community Preventive Services*; and the Health Technology Advisory Committee (HTAC) of the Minnesota Health Care Commission (MHCC) health technology evaluations.

Coffee Break: Tutorials for Biologists[37]

Some patients may wish to have access to a general healthcare site that takes a scientific view of the news and covers recent breakthroughs in biology that may one day assist physicians in developing treatments. To this end, we recommend "Coffee Break," a collection of short reports on recent biological discoveries. Each report incorporates interactive tutorials that demonstrate how bioinformatics tools are used as a part of the research process. Currently, all Coffee Breaks are written by NCBI staff.[38] Each report is about 400 words and is usually based on a discovery reported in one or more articles from recently published, peer-reviewed literature.[39] This site has new articles every few weeks, so it can be considered an online magazine of sorts, and intended for general background information. You can access the Coffee Break Web site at **http://www.ncbi.nlm.nih.gov/Coffeebreak/**.

Other Commercial Databases

In addition to resources maintained by official agencies, other databases exist that are commercial ventures addressing medical professionals. Here are a few examples that may interest you:

- **CliniWeb International:** Index and table of contents to selected clinical information on the Internet; see **http://www.ohsu.edu/cliniweb/**.

- **Image Engine:** Multimedia electronic medical record system that integrates a wide range of digitized clinical images with textual data stored in the University of Pittsburgh Medical Center's MARS electronic medical record system; see the following Web site: **http://www.cml.upmc.edu/cml/imageengine/imageEngine.html**.

- **Medical World Search:** Searches full text from thousands of selected medical sites on the Internet; see **http://www.mwsearch.com/**.

- **MedWeaver:** Prototype system that allows users to search differential diagnoses for any list of signs and symptoms and to search medical literature; see **http://www.med.virginia.edu/~wmd4n/medweaver.html**.

---

[37] Adapted from http://www.ncbi.nlm.nih.gov/Coffeebreak/Archive/FAQ.html.

[38] The figure that accompanies each article is frequently supplied by an expert external to NCBI, in which case the source of the figure is cited. The result is an interactive tutorial that tells a biological story.

[39] After a brief introduction that sets the work described into a broader context, the report focuses on how a molecular understanding can provide explanations of observed biology and lead to therapies for diseases. Each vignette is accompanied by a figure and hypertext links that lead to a series of pages that interactively show how NCBI tools and resources are used in the research process.

- **Metaphrase:** Middleware component intended for use by both caregivers and medical records personnel. It converts the informal language generally used by caregivers into terms from formal, controlled vocabularies; see **http://www.lexical.com/Metaphrase.html**.

The Genome Project and Sarcoidosis

With all the discussion in the press about the Human Genome Project, it is only natural that physicians, researchers, and patients want to know about how human genes relate to sarcoidosis. In the following section, we will discuss databases and references used by physicians and scientists who work in this area.

Online Mendelian Inheritance in Man (OMIM)

The Online Mendelian Inheritance in Man (OMIM) database is a catalog of human genes and genetic disorders authored and edited by Dr. Victor A. McKusick and his colleagues at Johns Hopkins and elsewhere. OMIM was developed for the World Wide Web by the National Center for Biotechnology Information (NCBI).[40] The database contains textual information, pictures, and reference information. It also contains copious links to NCBI's Entrez database of MEDLINE articles and sequence information.

Go to **http://www.ncbi.nlm.nih.gov/Omim/searchomim.html** to search the database. Type "sarcoidosis" (or synonyms) in the search box, and click "Submit Search." If too many results appear, you can narrow the search by adding the word "clinical." Each report will have additional links to related research and databases. By following these links, especially the link titled "Database Links," you will be exposed to numerous specialized databases that are largely used by the scientific community. These databases are overly technical and seldom used by the general public, but offer an abundance of information. The following is an example of the results you can obtain from the OMIM for sarcoidosis:

---

[40] Adapted from **http://www.ncbi.nlm.nih.gov/**. Established in 1988 as a national resource for molecular biology information, NCBI creates public databases, conducts research in computational biology, develops software tools for analyzing genome data, and disseminates biomedical information--all for the better understanding of molecular processes affecting human health and disease.

- **Sarcoidosis**
  Web site: http://www.ncbi.nlm.nih.gov/htbin-post/Omim/dispmim?181000

Genes and Disease (NCBI - Map)

The Genes and Disease database is produced by the National Center for Biotechnology Information of the National Library of Medicine at the National Institutes of Health. Go to **http://www.ncbi.nlm.nih.gov/disease/**, and browse the system pages to have a full view of important conditions linked to human genes. Since this site is regularly updated, you may wish to re-visit it from time to time. The following systems and associated disorders are addressed:

- **Metabolism:** Food and energy.
  Examples: Adreno-leukodystrophy, Atherosclerosis, Best disease, Gaucher disease, Glucose galactose malabsorption, Gyrate atrophy, Juvenile onset diabetes, Obesity, Paroxysmal nocturnal hemoglobinuria, Phenylketonuria, Refsum disease, Tangier disease, Tay-Sachs disease.
  Web site: **http://www.ncbi.nlm.nih.gov/disease/Metabolism.html**

- **Muscle and Bone:** Movement and growth.
  Examples: Duchenne muscular dystrophy, Ellis-van Creveld syndrome, Marfan syndrome, myotonic dystrophy, spinal muscular atrophy.
  Web site: **http://www.ncbi.nlm.nih.gov/disease/Muscle.html**

- **Nervous System:** Mind and body.
  Examples: Alzheimer disease, Amyotrophic lateral sclerosis, Angelman syndrome, Charcot-Marie-Tooth disease, epilepsy, essential tremor, Fragile X syndrome, Friedreich's ataxia, Huntington disease, Niemann-Pick disease, Parkinson disease, Prader-Willi syndrome, Rett syndrome, Spinocerebellar atrophy, Williams syndrome.
  Web site: **http://www.ncbi.nlm.nih.gov/disease/Brain.html**

- **Signals:** Cellular messages.
  Examples: Ataxia telangiectasia, Baldness, Cockayne syndrome, Glaucoma, SRY: sex determination, Tuberous sclerosis, Waardenburg syndrome, Werner syndrome.
  Web site: **http://www.ncbi.nlm.nih.gov/disease/Signals.html**

- **Transporters:** Pumps and channels.
  Examples: Cystic Fibrosis, deafness, diastrophic dysplasia, Hemophilia A, long-QT syndrome, Menkes syndrome, Pendred syndrome, polycystic kidney disease, sickle cell anemia, Wilson's disease, Zellweger syndrome.
  Web site: **http://www.ncbi.nlm.nih.gov/disease/Transporters.html**

Entrez

Entrez is a search and retrieval system that integrates several linked databases at the National Center for Biotechnology Information (NCBI). These databases include nucleotide sequences, protein sequences, macromolecular structures, whole genomes, and MEDLINE through PubMed. Entrez provides access to the following databases:

- **PubMed:** Biomedical literature (PubMed),
  Web site: **http://www.ncbi.nlm.nih.gov/entrez/query.fcgi?db=PubMed**

- **Nucleotide Sequence Database (Genbank):**
  Web site:
  http://www.ncbi.nlm.nih.gov/entrez/query.fcgi?db=Nucleotide

- **Protein Sequence Database:**
  Web site: **http://www.ncbi.nlm.nih.gov/entrez/query.fcgi?db=Protein**

- **Structure:** Three-dimensional macromolecular structures,
  Web site: **http://www.ncbi.nlm.nih.gov/entrez/query.fcgi?db=Structure**

- **Genome:** Complete genome assemblies,
  Web site: **http://www.ncbi.nlm.nih.gov/entrez/query.fcgi?db=Genome**

- **PopSet:** Population study data sets,
  Web site: **http://www.ncbi.nlm.nih.gov/entrez/query.fcgi?db=Popset**

- **OMIM:** Online Mendelian Inheritance in Man,
  Web site: **http://www.ncbi.nlm.nih.gov/entrez/query.fcgi?db=OMIM**

- **Taxonomy:** Organisms in GenBank,
  Web site:
  http://www.ncbi.nlm.nih.gov/entrez/query.fcgi?db=Taxonomy

- **Books:** Online books,
  Web site: **http://www.ncbi.nlm.nih.gov/entrez/query.fcgi?db=books**

- **ProbeSet:** Gene Expression Omnibus (GEO),
  Web site: **http://www.ncbi.nlm.nih.gov/entrez/query.fcgi?db=geo**

- **3D Domains:** Domains from Entrez Structure,
  Web site: **http://www.ncbi.nlm.nih.gov/entrez/query.fcgi?db=geo**

- **NCBI's Protein Sequence Information Survey Results:**
  Web site: **http://www.ncbi.nlm.nih.gov/About/proteinsurvey/**

To access the Entrez system at the National Center for Biotechnology Information, go to **http://www.ncbi.nlm.nih.gov/entrez**, and then select the database that you would like to search. The databases available are listed in the drop box next to "Search." In the box next to "for," enter "sarcoidosis" (or synonyms) and click "Go."

Jablonski's Multiple Congenital Anomaly/Mental Retardation (MCA/MR) Syndromes Database[41]

This online resource can be quite useful. It has been developed to facilitate the identification and differentiation of syndromic entities. Special attention is given to the type of information that is usually limited or completely omitted in existing reference sources due to space limitations of the printed form.

At **http://www.nlm.nih.gov/mesh/jablonski/syndrome_toc/toc_a.html** you can also search across syndromes using an alphabetical index. You can also search at **http://www.nlm.nih.gov/mesh/jablonski/syndrome_db.html**.

The Genome Database[42]

Established at Johns Hopkins University in Baltimore, Maryland in 1990, the Genome Database (GDB) is the official central repository for genomic mapping data resulting from the Human Genome Initiative. In the spring of 1999, the Bioinformatics Supercomputing Centre (BiSC) at the Hospital for Sick Children in Toronto, Ontario assumed the management of GDB. The Human Genome Initiative is a worldwide research effort focusing on structural analysis of human DNA to determine the location and sequence of the estimated 100,000 human genes. In support of this project, GDB stores and curates data generated by researchers worldwide who are engaged in the mapping effort of the Human Genome Project (HGP). GDB's mission is to provide scientists with an encyclopedia of the human genome which is continually revised and updated to reflect the current state of scientific knowledge. Although GDB has historically focused on gene mapping, its focus will broaden as the Genome Project moves from mapping to sequence, and finally, to functional analysis.

To access the GDB, simply go to the following hyperlink: **http://www.gdb.org/**. Search "All Biological Data" by "Keyword." Type "sarcoidosis" (or synonyms) into the search box, and review the results. If

---

[41] Adapted from the National Library of Medicine: http://www.nlm.nih.gov/mesh/jablonski/about_syndrome.html.
[42] Adapted from the Genome Database: **http://gdbwww.gdb.org/gdb/aboutGDB.html#mission**.

more than one word is used in the search box, then separate each one with the word "and" or "or" (using "or" might be useful when using synonyms). This database is extremely technical as it was created for specialists. The articles are the results which are the most accessible to non-professionals and often listed under the heading "Citations." The contact names are also accessible to non-professionals.

Specialized References

The following books are specialized references written for professionals interested in sarcoidosis (sorted alphabetically by title, hyperlinks provide rankings, information, and reviews at Amazon.com):

- **Atlas of Lung Pathology**; Hardcover, Cd-Rom edition (July 1997), Lippincott Williams & Wilkins Publishers; ISBN: 0412112116; http://www.amazon.com/exec/obidos/ASIN/0412112116/icongroupinterna

- **Differential Diagnosis in Pathology: Pulmonary Disorders (Differential Diagnosis in Pathology)** by Anthony A. Gal, M.D., Michael N. Koss, M.D.; Hardcover (August 1997), Lippincott, Williams & Wilkins; ISBN: 0683303015; http://www.amazon.com/exec/obidos/ASIN/0683303015/icongroupinterna

- **Foundations of Respiratory Care** by Kenneth A. Wyka, William F. Clark, Paul J. Mathews; Hardcover - 1032 pages, 1st edition (January 15, 2002), Delmar Learning; ISBN: 0766808939; http://www.amazon.com/exec/obidos/ASIN/0766808939/icongroupinterna

- **Lung Disorders Sourcebook** by Dawn D. Matthews; Hardcover, 1st edition (March 2002), Omnigraphics, Inc.; ISBN: 0780803396; http://www.amazon.com/exec/obidos/ASIN/0780803396/icongroupinterna

- **Pulmonary Diseases and Disorders Companion Handbook** by Alfred P. Fishman; Paperback, 3rd edition (April 15, 2002), McGraw-Hill; ISBN: 0070220026; http://www.amazon.com/exec/obidos/ASIN/0070220026/icongroupinterna

- **Textbook of Respiratory Medicine (Two-Volume Set)** by John F. Murray, Jay A. Nadel; Hardcover - 2562 pages, 3rd edition (May 15, 2000), W B Saunders Co; ISBN: 0721677118; http://www.amazon.com/exec/obidos/ASIN/0721677118/icongroupinterna

CHAPTER 10. DISSERTATIONS ON SARCOIDOSIS

Overview

University researchers are active in studying almost all known diseases. The result of research is often published in the form of Doctoral or Master's dissertations. You should understand, therefore, that applied diagnostic procedures and/or therapies can take many years to develop after the thesis that proposed the new technique or approach was written.

In this chapter, we will give you a bibliography on recent dissertations relating to sarcoidosis. You can read about these in more detail using the Internet or your local medical library. We will also provide you with information on how to use the Internet to stay current on dissertations.

Dissertations on Sarcoidosis

ProQuest Digital Dissertations is the largest archive of academic dissertations available. From this archive, we have compiled the following list covering dissertations devoted to sarcoidosis. You will see that the information provided includes the dissertation's title, its author, and the author's institution. To read more about the following, simply use the Internet address indicated. The following covers recent dissertations dealing with sarcoidosis:

- **Molecular Cloning and Functional Analysis of the Human Interleukin-16 Gene** by Mukhtar, Abdu Sarkinbai; Phd from Boston University, 2000, 197 pages
  http://wwwlib.umi.com/dissertations/fullcit/9942396

Keeping Current

As previously mentioned, an effective way to stay current on dissertations dedicated to sarcoidosis is to use the database called *ProQuest Digital Dissertations* via the Internet, located at the following Web address: **http://wwwlib.umi.com/dissertations.** The site allows you to freely access the last two years of citations and abstracts. Ask your medical librarian if the library has full and unlimited access to this database. From the library, you should be able to do more complete searches than with the limited 2-year access available to the general public.

PART III. APPENDICES

ABOUT PART III

Part III is a collection of appendices on general medical topics which may be of interest to patients with sarcoidosis and related conditions.

APPENDIX A. RESEARCHING YOUR MEDICATIONS

Overview

There are a number of sources available on new or existing medications which could be prescribed to patients with sarcoidosis. While a number of hard copy or CD-Rom resources are available to patients and physicians for research purposes, a more flexible method is to use Internet-based databases. In this chapter, we will begin with a general overview of medications. We will then proceed to outline official recommendations on how you should view your medications. You may also want to research medications that you are currently taking for other conditions as they may interact with medications for sarcoidosis. Research can give you information on the side effects, interactions, and limitations of prescription drugs used in the treatment of sarcoidosis. Broadly speaking, there are two sources of information on approved medications: public sources and private sources. We will emphasize free-to-use public sources.

Your Medications: The Basics[43]

The Agency for Health Care Research and Quality has published extremely useful guidelines on how you can best participate in the medication aspects of sarcoidosis. Taking medicines is not always as simple as swallowing a pill. It can involve many steps and decisions each day. The AHCRQ recommends that patients with sarcoidosis take part in treatment decisions. Do not be afraid to ask questions and talk about your concerns. By taking a moment to ask questions early, you may avoid problems later. Here are some points to cover each time a new medicine is prescribed:

- Ask about all parts of your treatment, including diet changes, exercise, and medicines.

- Ask about the risks and benefits of each medicine or other treatment you might receive.

- Ask how often you or your doctor will check for side effects from a given medication.

Do not hesitate to ask what is important to you about your medicines. You may want a medicine with the fewest side effects, or the fewest doses to take each day. You may care most about cost, or how the medicine might affect how you live or work. Or, you may want the medicine your doctor believes will work the best. Telling your doctor will help him or her select the best treatment for you.

Do not be afraid to "bother" your doctor with your concerns and questions about medications for sarcoidosis. You can also talk to a nurse or a pharmacist. They can help you better understand your treatment plan. Feel free to bring a friend or family member with you when you visit your doctor. Talking over your options with someone you trust can help you make better choices, especially if you are not feeling well. Specifically, ask your doctor the following:

- The name of the medicine and what it is supposed to do.

- How and when to take the medicine, how much to take, and for how long.

- What food, drinks, other medicines, or activities you should avoid while taking the medicine.

- What side effects the medicine may have, and what to do if they occur.

---

[43] This section is adapted from AHCRQ: **http://www.ahcpr.gov/consumer/ncpiebro.htm** .

- If you can get a refill, and how often.

- About any terms or directions you do not understand.

- What to do if you miss a dose.

- If there is written information you can take home (most pharmacies have information sheets on your prescription medicines; some even offer large-print or Spanish versions).

Do not forget to tell your doctor about all the medicines you are currently taking (not just those for sarcoidosis). This includes prescription medicines and the medicines that you buy over the counter. Then your doctor can avoid giving you a new medicine that may not work well with the medications you take now. When talking to your doctor, you may wish to prepare a list of medicines you currently take, the reason you take them, and how you take them. Be sure to include the following information for each:

- Name of medicine

- Reason taken

- Dosage

- Time(s) of day

Also include any over-the-counter medicines, such as:

- Laxatives

- Diet pills

- Vitamins

- Cold medicine

- Aspirin or other pain, headache, or fever medicine

- Cough medicine

- Allergy relief medicine

- Antacids

- Sleeping pills

- Others (include names)

Learning More about Your Medications

Because of historical investments by various organizations and the emergence of the Internet, it has become rather simple to learn about the medications your doctor has recommended for sarcoidosis. One such source is the United States Pharmacopeia. In 1820, eleven physicians met in Washington, D.C. to establish the first compendium of standard drugs for the United States. They called this compendium the "U.S. Pharmacopeia (USP)." Today, the USP is a non-profit organization consisting of 800 volunteer scientists, eleven elected officials, and 400 representatives of state associations and colleges of medicine and pharmacy. The USP is located in Rockville, Maryland, and its home page is located at **www.usp.org**. The USP currently provides standards for over 3,700 medications. The resulting USP DI® Advice for the Patient® can be accessed through the National Library of Medicine of the National Institutes of Health. The database is partially derived from lists of federally approved medications in the Food and Drug Administration's (FDA) Drug Approvals database.[44]

While the FDA database is rather large and difficult to navigate, the Phamacopeia is both user-friendly and free to use. It covers more than 9,000 prescription and over-the-counter medications. To access this database, simply type the following hyperlink into your Web browser: **http://www.nlm.nih.gov/medlineplus/druginformation.html**. To view examples of a given medication (brand names, category, description, preparation, proper use, precautions, side effects, etc.), simply follow the hyperlinks indicated within the United States Pharmacopoeia. It is important to read the disclaimer by the United States Pharmacopoeia (**http://www.nlm.nih.gov/medlineplus/drugdisclaimer.html**) before using the information provided.

Of course, we as editors cannot be certain as to what medications you are taking. Therefore, we have compiled a list of medications associated with the treatment of sarcoidosis. Once again, due to space limitations, we only list a sample of medications and provide hyperlinks to ample documentation (e.g. typical dosage, side effects, drug-interaction risks, etc.). The following drugs have been mentioned in the Pharmacopeia and other sources as being potentially applicable to sarcoidosis:

---

[44] Though cumbersome, the FDA database can be freely browsed at the following site: **www.fda.gov/cder/da/da.htm**.

Azathioprine

- **Systemic - U.S. Brands:** Imuran
  http://www.nlm.nih.gov/medlineplus/druginfo/azathioprinesys
  temic202077.html

Chlorambucil

- **Systemic - U.S. Brands:** Leukeran
  http://www.nlm.nih.gov/medlineplus/druginfo/chlorambucilsys
  temic202124.html

Chloroquine

- **Systemic - U.S. Brands:** Aralen
  http://www.nlm.nih.gov/medlineplus/druginfo/chloroquinesyst
  emic202133.html

Corticosteroids

- **Dental - U.S. Brands:** Kenalog in Orabase; Orabase-HCA; Oracort;
  Oralone
  http://www.nlm.nih.gov/medlineplus/druginfo/corticosteroidsd
  ental202010.html
- **Inhalation - U.S. Brands:** AeroBid; AeroBid-M; Azmacort;
  Beclovent; Decadron Respihaler; Pulmicort Respules; Pulmicort
  Turbuhaler; Vanceril; Vanceril 84 mcg Double Strength
  http://www.nlm.nih.gov/medlineplus/druginfo/corticosteroidsi
  nhalation202011.html
- **Nasal - U.S. Brands:** Beconase; Beconase AQ; Dexacort Turbinaire;
  Flonase; Nasacort; Nasacort AQ; Nasalide; Nasarel; Nasonex;
  Rhinocort; Vancenase; Vancenase AQ 84 mcg; Vancenase
  pockethaler
  http://www.nlm.nih.gov/medlineplus/druginfo/corticosteroidsn
  asal202012.html
- **Ophthalmic - U.S. Brands:** AK-Dex; AK-Pred; AK-Tate; Baldex;
  Decadron; Dexair; Dexotic; Econopred; Econopred Plus; Eflone;
  Flarex; Fluor-Op; FML Forte; FML Liquifilm; FML S.O.P.; HMS
  Liquifilm; Inflamase Forte; Inflamase Mild; I-Pred; Lite Pred;
  Maxidex; Ocu-Dex; Ocu-Pred; Ocu-Pr
  http://www.nlm.nih.gov/medlineplus/druginfo/corticosteroidso
  phthalmic202013.html
- **Otic - U.S. Brands:** Decadron
  http://www.nlm.nih.gov/medlineplus/druginfo/corticosteroidso
  tic202014.html

- **Rectal - U.S. Brands:** Anucort-HC; Anu-Med HC; Anuprep HC; Anusol-HC; Anutone-HC; Anuzone-HC; Cort-Dome; Cortenema; Cortifoam; Hemorrhoidal HC; Hemril-HC Uniserts; Proctocort; Proctosol-HC; Rectosol-HC
  http://www.nlm.nih.gov/medlineplus/druginfo/corticosteroidsrectal203366.html

Cyclophosphamide

- **Systemic - U.S. Brands:** Cytoxan; Neosar
  http://www.nlm.nih.gov/medlineplus/druginfo/cyclophosphamidesystemic202174.html

Hydroxychloroquine

- **Systemic - U.S. Brands:** Plaquenil
  http://www.nlm.nih.gov/medlineplus/druginfo/hydroxychloroquinesystemic202288.html

Thalidomide

- **Systemic - U.S. Brands:** THALOMID
  http://www.nlm.nih.gov/medlineplus/druginfo/thalidomidesystemic202692.html

Commercial Databases

In addition to the medications listed in the USP above, a number of commercial sites are available by subscription to physicians and their institutions. You may be able to access these sources from your local medical library or your doctor's office.

Reuters Health Drug Database

The Reuters Health Drug Database can be searched by keyword at the hyperlink: **http://www.reutershealth.com/frame2/drug.html**. The following medications are listed in the Reuters' database as associated with sarcoidosis (including those with contraindications):[45]

- **Chloroquine**
  http://www.reutershealth.com/atoz/html/Chloroquine.htm

---

[45] Adapted from *A to Z Drug Facts* by Facts and Comparisons.

- **Cyclosporine**
  http://www.reutershealth.com/atoz/html/Cyclosporine.htm

- **Cyclosporine(Cyclosporin A)**
  http://www.reutershealth.com/atoz/html/Cyclosporine(Cyclosporin_A).htm

- **Estradiol**
  http://www.reutershealth.com/atoz/html/Estradiol.htm

- **Estrogens Conjugated**
  http://www.reutershealth.com/atoz/html/Estrogens_Conjugated.htm

- **Estropipate**
  http://www.reutershealth.com/atoz/html/Estropipate.htm

- **Estropipate (Piperazine Estrone Sulfate)**
  http://www.reutershealth.com/atoz/html/Estropipate_(Piperazine_Estrone_Sulfate).htm

- **Methimazole**
  http://www.reutershealth.com/atoz/html/Methimazole.htm

- **Nevirapine**
  http://www.reutershealth.com/atoz/html/Nevirapine.htm

- **Propylthiouracil**
  http://www.reutershealth.com/atoz/html/Propylthiouracil.htm

- **Thalidomide**
  http://www.reutershealth.com/atoz/html/Thalidomide.htm

- **Tuberculin Purified Protein Derivative**
  http://www.reutershealth.com/atoz/html/Tuberculin_Purified_Protein_Derivative.htm

Mosby's GenRx

Mosby's GenRx database (also available on CD-Rom and book format) covers 45,000 drug products including generics and international brands. It provides prescribing information, drug interactions, and patient information. Information in Mosby's GenRx database can be obtained at the following hyperlink: **http://www.genrx.com/Mosby/PhyGenRx/group.html**.

Physicians Desk Reference

The Physicians Desk Reference database (also available in CD-Rom and book format) is a full-text drug database. The database is searchable by brand name, generic name or by indication. It features multiple drug interactions reports. Information can be obtained at the following hyperlink: **http://physician.pdr.net/physician/templates/en/acl/psuser_t.htm**.

Other Web Sites

A number of additional Web sites discuss drug information. As an example, you may like to look at **www.drugs.com** which reproduces the information in the Pharmacopeia as well as commercial information. You may also want to consider the Web site of the Medical Letter, Inc. which allows users to download articles on various drugs and therapeutics for a nominal fee: **http://www.medletter.com/**.

Contraindications and Interactions (Hidden Dangers)

Some of the medications mentioned in the previous discussions can be problematic for patients with sarcoidosis--not because they are used in the treatment process, but because of contraindications, or side effects. Medications with contraindications are those that could react with drugs used to treat sarcoidosis or potentially create deleterious side effects in patients with sarcoidosis. You should ask your physician about any contraindications, especially as these might apply to other medications that you may be taking for common ailments.

Drug-drug interactions occur when two or more drugs react with each other. This drug-drug interaction may cause you to experience an unexpected side effect. Drug interactions may make your medications less effective, cause unexpected side effects, or increase the action of a particular drug. Some drug interactions can even be harmful to you.

Be sure to read the label every time you use a nonprescription or prescription drug, and take the time to learn about drug interactions. These precautions may be critical to your health. You can reduce the risk of potentially harmful drug interactions and side effects with a little bit of knowledge and common sense.

Drug labels contain important information about ingredients, uses, warnings, and directions which you should take the time to read and understand. Labels also include warnings about possible drug interactions. Further, drug labels may change as new information becomes available. This is why it's especially important to read the label every time you use a medication. When your doctor prescribes a new drug, discuss all over-the-counter and prescription medications, dietary supplements, vitamins, botanicals, minerals and herbals you take as well as the foods you eat. Ask your pharmacist for the package insert for each prescription drug you take. The package insert provides more information about potential drug interactions.

A Final Warning

At some point, you may hear of alternative medications from friends, relatives, or in the news media. Advertisements may suggest that certain alternative drugs can produce positive results for patients with sarcoidosis. Exercise caution--some of these drugs may have fraudulent claims, and others may actually hurt you. The Food and Drug Administration (FDA) is the official U.S. agency charged with discovering which medications are likely to improve the health of patients with sarcoidosis. The FDA warns patients to watch out for[46]:

- Secret formulas (real scientists share what they know)

- Amazing breakthroughs or miracle cures (real breakthroughs don't happen very often; when they do, real scientists do not call them amazing or miracles)

- Quick, painless, or guaranteed cures

- If it sounds too good to be true, it probably isn't true.

If you have any questions about any kind of medical treatment, the FDA may have an office near you. Look for their number in the blue pages of the phone book. You can also contact the FDA through its toll-free number, 1-888-INFO-FDA (1-888-463-6332), or on the World Wide Web at **www.fda.gov**.

---

[46] This section has been adapted from **http://www.fda.gov/opacom/lowlit/medfraud.html**

General References

In addition to the resources provided earlier in this chapter, the following general references describe medications (sorted alphabetically by title; hyperlinks provide rankings, information and reviews at Amazon.com):

- **Delmar's Respiratory Care Drug Reference** by Fred Hill; Paperback - 575 pages, 1st edition (January 15, 1999), Delmar Learning; ISBN: 0827390661; **http://www.amazon.com/exec/obidos/ASIN/0827390661/icongroupinterna**

- **Mosby's Respiratory Care Drug Reference** by Joseph L., Jr. Rau; Paperback - 352 pages, 1st edition (January 15, 1997), Mosby-Year Book; ISBN: 0815184565; **http://www.amazon.com/exec/obidos/ASIN/0815184565/icongroupinterna**

- **Pharmacology in Respiratory Care** by Stuart R. Levine, Henry Hitner, Arthur J. McLaughlin, Jr.; Hardcover - 386 pages (May 11, 2001), Appleton & Lange; ISBN: 0071347275; **http://www.amazon.com/exec/obidos/ASIN/0071347275/icongroupinterna**

- **Respiratory Care Drug Reference** by Arthur McLaughlin; Paperback - 383 pages, 2 edition (March 1997), Unknown; ISBN: 0834207885; **http://www.amazon.com/exec/obidos/ASIN/0834207885/icongroupinterna**

Vocabulary Builder

The following vocabulary builder gives definitions of words used in this chapter that have not been defined in previous chapters:

Estradiol: The most potent mammalian estrogenic hormone. It is produced in the ovary, placenta, testis, and possibly the adrenal cortex. [NIH]

Inhalation: The drawing of air or other substances into the lungs. [EU]

Liquifilm: A thin liquid layer of coating. [EU]

Methimazole: A thioureylene antithyroid agent that inhibits the formation of thyroid hormones by interfering with the incorporation of iodine into tyrosyl residues of thyroglobulin. This is done by interfering with the oxidation of iodide ion and iodotyrosyl groups through inhibition of the peroxidase enzyme. [NIH]

Nevirapine: A potent, non-nucleoside reverse transcriptase inhibitor used in combination with nucleoside analogues for treatment of HIV infection and AIDS. [NIH]

Rectal: Pertaining to the rectum (= distal portion of the large intestine). [EU]

APPENDIX B. RESEARCHING ALTERNATIVE MEDICINE

Overview

Complementary and alternative medicine (CAM) is one of the most contentious aspects of modern medical practice. You may have heard of these treatments on the radio or on television. Maybe you have seen articles written about these treatments in magazines, newspapers, or books. Perhaps your friends or doctor have mentioned alternatives.

In this chapter, we will begin by giving you a broad perspective on complementary and alternative therapies. Next, we will introduce you to official information sources on CAM relating to sarcoidosis. Finally, at the conclusion of this chapter, we will provide a list of readings on sarcoidosis from various authors. We will begin, however, with the National Center for Complementary and Alternative Medicine's (NCCAM) overview of complementary and alternative medicine.

What Is CAM?[47]

Complementary and alternative medicine (CAM) covers a broad range of healing philosophies, approaches, and therapies. Generally, it is defined as those treatments and healthcare practices which are not taught in medical schools, used in hospitals, or reimbursed by medical insurance companies. Many CAM therapies are termed "holistic," which generally means that the healthcare practitioner considers the whole person, including physical, mental, emotional, and spiritual health. Some of these therapies are also known as "preventive," which means that the practitioner educates and

---

[47] Adapted from the NCCAM: **http://nccam.nih.gov/nccam/fcp/faq/index.html#what-is**.

treats the person to prevent health problems from arising, rather than treating symptoms after problems have occurred.

People use CAM treatments and therapies in a variety of ways. Therapies are used alone (often referred to as alternative), in combination with other alternative therapies, or in addition to conventional treatment (sometimes referred to as complementary). Complementary and alternative medicine, or "integrative medicine," includes a broad range of healing philosophies, approaches, and therapies. Some approaches are consistent with physiological principles of Western medicine, while others constitute healing systems with non-Western origins. While some therapies are far outside the realm of accepted Western medical theory and practice, others are becoming established in mainstream medicine.

Complementary and alternative therapies are used in an effort to prevent illness, reduce stress, prevent or reduce side effects and symptoms, or control or cure disease. Some commonly used methods of complementary or alternative therapy include mind/body control interventions such as visualization and relaxation, manual healing including acupressure and massage, homeopathy, vitamins or herbal products, and acupuncture.

What Are the Domains of Alternative Medicine?[48]

The list of CAM practices changes continually. The reason being is that these new practices and therapies are often proved to be safe and effective, and therefore become generally accepted as "mainstream" healthcare practices. Today, CAM practices may be grouped within five major domains: (1) alternative medical systems, (2) mind-body interventions, (3) biologically-based treatments, (4) manipulative and body-based methods, and (5) energy therapies. The individual systems and treatments comprising these categories are too numerous to list in this sourcebook. Thus, only limited examples are provided within each.

Alternative Medical Systems

Alternative medical systems involve complete systems of theory and practice that have evolved independent of, and often prior to, conventional biomedical approaches. Many are traditional systems of medicine that are

---

[48] Adapted from the NCCAM: http://nccam.nih.gov/nccam/fcp/classify/index.html.

practiced by individual cultures throughout the world, including a number of venerable Asian approaches.

Traditional oriental medicine emphasizes the balance or disturbances of qi (pronounced chi) or vital energy in health and disease, respectively. Traditional oriental medicine consists of a group of techniques and methods including acupuncture, herbal medicine, oriental massage, and qi gong (a form of energy therapy). Acupuncture involves stimulating specific anatomic points in the body for therapeutic purposes, usually by puncturing the skin with a thin needle.

Ayurveda is India's traditional system of medicine. Ayurvedic medicine (meaning "science of life") is a comprehensive system of medicine that places equal emphasis on body, mind, and spirit. Ayurveda strives to restore the innate harmony of the individual. Some of the primary Ayurvedic treatments include diet, exercise, meditation, herbs, massage, exposure to sunlight, and controlled breathing.

Other traditional healing systems have been developed by the world's indigenous populations. These populations include Native American, Aboriginal, African, Middle Eastern, Tibetan, and Central and South American cultures. Homeopathy and naturopathy are also examples of complete alternative medicine systems.

Homeopathic medicine is an unconventional Western system that is based on the principle that "like cures like," i.e., that the same substance that in large doses produces the symptoms of an illness, in very minute doses cures it. Homeopathic health practitioners believe that the more dilute the remedy, the greater its potency. Therefore, they use small doses of specially prepared plant extracts and minerals to stimulate the body's defense mechanisms and healing processes in order to treat illness.

Naturopathic medicine is based on the theory that disease is a manifestation of alterations in the processes by which the body naturally heals itself and emphasizes health restoration rather than disease treatment. Naturopathic physicians employ an array of healing practices, including the following: diet and clinical nutrition, homeopathy, acupuncture, herbal medicine, hydrotherapy (the use of water in a range of temperatures and methods of applications), spinal and soft-tissue manipulation, physical therapies (such as those involving electrical currents, ultrasound, and light), therapeutic counseling, and pharmacology.

Mind-Body Interventions

Mind-body interventions employ a variety of techniques designed to facilitate the mind's capacity to affect bodily function and symptoms. Only a select group of mind-body interventions having well-documented theoretical foundations are considered CAM. For example, patient education and cognitive-behavioral approaches are now considered "mainstream." On the other hand, complementary and alternative medicine includes meditation, certain uses of hypnosis, dance, music, and art therapy, as well as prayer and mental healing.

Biological-Based Therapies

This category of CAM includes natural and biological-based practices, interventions, and products, many of which overlap with conventional medicine's use of dietary supplements. This category includes herbal, special dietary, orthomolecular, and individual biological therapies.

Herbal therapy employs an individual herb or a mixture of herbs for healing purposes. An herb is a plant or plant part that produces and contains chemical substances that act upon the body. Special diet therapies, such as those proposed by Drs. Atkins, Ornish, Pritikin, and Weil, are believed to prevent and/or control illness as well as promote health. Orthomolecular therapies aim to treat disease with varying concentrations of chemicals such as magnesium, melatonin, and mega-doses of vitamins. Biological therapies include, for example, the use of laetrile and shark cartilage to treat cancer and the use of bee pollen to treat autoimmune and inflammatory diseases.

Manipulative and Body-Based Methods

This category includes methods that are based on manipulation and/or movement of the body. For example, chiropractors focus on the relationship between structure and function, primarily pertaining to the spine, and how that relationship affects the preservation and restoration of health. Chiropractors use manipulative therapy as an integral treatment tool.

In contrast, osteopaths place particular emphasis on the musculoskeletal system and practice osteopathic manipulation. Osteopaths believe that all of the body's systems work together and that disturbances in one system may have an impact upon function elsewhere in the body. Massage therapists manipulate the soft tissues of the body to normalize those tissues.

Energy Therapies

Energy therapies focus on energy fields originating within the body (biofields) or those from other sources (electromagnetic fields). Biofield therapies are intended to affect energy fields (the existence of which is not yet experimentally proven) that surround and penetrate the human body. Some forms of energy therapy manipulate biofields by applying pressure and/or manipulating the body by placing the hands in or through these fields. Examples include Qi gong, Reiki and Therapeutic Touch.

Qi gong is a component of traditional oriental medicine that combines movement, meditation, and regulation of breathing to enhance the flow of vital energy (qi) in the body, improve blood circulation, and enhance immune function. Reiki, the Japanese word representing Universal Life Energy, is based on the belief that, by channeling spiritual energy through the practitioner, the spirit is healed and, in turn, heals the physical body. Therapeutic Touch is derived from the ancient technique of "laying-on of hands." It is based on the premises that the therapist's healing force affects the patient's recovery and that healing is promoted when the body's energies are in balance. By passing their hands over the patient, these healers identify energy imbalances.

Bioelectromagnetic-based therapies involve the unconventional use of electromagnetic fields to treat illnesses or manage pain. These therapies are often used to treat asthma, cancer, and migraine headaches. Types of electromagnetic fields which are manipulated in these therapies include pulsed fields, magnetic fields, and alternating current or direct current fields.

Can Alternatives Affect My Treatment?

A critical issue in pursuing complementary alternatives mentioned thus far is the risk that these might have undesirable interactions with your medical treatment. It becomes all the more important to speak with your doctor who can offer advice on the use of alternatives. Official sources confirm this view. Though written for women, we find that the National Women's Health Information Center's advice on pursuing alternative medicine is appropriate for patients of both genders and all ages.[49]

---

[49] Adapted from **http://www.4woman.gov/faq/alternative.htm**.

Is It Okay to Want Both Traditional and Alternative Medicine?

Should you wish to explore non-traditional types of treatment, be sure to discuss all issues concerning treatments and therapies with your healthcare provider, whether a physician or practitioner of complementary and alternative medicine. Competent healthcare management requires knowledge of both conventional and alternative therapies you are taking for the practitioner to have a complete picture of your treatment plan.

The decision to use complementary and alternative treatments is an important one. Consider before selecting an alternative therapy, the safety and effectiveness of the therapy or treatment, the expertise and qualifications of the healthcare practitioner, and the quality of delivery. These topics should be considered when selecting any practitioner or therapy.

Finding CAM References on Sarcoidosis

Having read the previous discussion, you may be wondering which complementary or alternative treatments might be appropriate for sarcoidosis. For the remainder of this chapter, we will direct you to a number of official sources which can assist you in researching studies and publications. Some of these articles are rather technical, so some patience may be required.

The Combined Health Information Database

For a targeted search, The Combined Health Information Database is a bibliographic database produced by health-related agencies of the Federal Government (mostly from the National Institutes of Health). This database is updated four times a year at the end of January, April, July, and October. Check the titles, summaries, and availability of CAM-related information by using the "Simple Search" option at the following Web site: **http://chid.nih.gov/simple/simple.html**. In the drop box at the top, select "Complementary and Alternative Medicine." Then type "sarcoidosis" (or synonyms) in the second search box. We recommend that you select 100 "documents per page" and to check the "whole records" options. The following was extracted using this technique:

- **Improvements in Chronic Diseases With a Comprehensive Natural Medicine Approach: A Review and Case Series**

  Source: Behavioral Medicine. 26(1): 34-46. Spring 2000.

Summary: This journal article presents a case series describing the use of Maharishi Vedic Medicine (MVM) for the treatment of chronic disorders. According to the authors, many reports suggest health benefits from individual MVM techniques. However, reports on integrated holistic approaches are rare. This case series is designed to investigate the effectiveness of an integrated, multimodality MVM program during a 3-week period of residential treatment followed by 3 months of home-based care. The key components of the program included transcendental meditation, pulse diagnosis, Vedic sound therapy, a traditional Vedic medicine diet, herbal preparations, physiological purification procedures, Vedic exercise, and environmental analyses. This article describes the outcomes in four patients: one with sarcoidosis; one with Parkinson's disease; one with renal hypertension; and one with diabetes mellitus, essential hypertension, and anxiety disorder. Results suggested substantial improvements as indicated by reductions in major signs, symptoms, and use of conventional medicines in all four patients. The article has 4 tables and 82 references.

National Center for Complementary and Alternative Medicine

The National Center for Complementary and Alternative Medicine (NCCAM) of the National Institutes of Health (http://nccam.nih.gov) has created a link to the National Library of Medicine's databases to allow patients to search for articles that specifically relate to sarcoidosis and complementary medicine. To search the database, go to the following Web site: **www.nlm.nih.gov/nccam/camonpubmed.html**. Select "CAM on PubMed." Enter "sarcoidosis" (or synonyms) into the search box. Click "Go." The following references provide information on particular aspects of complementary and alternative medicine (CAM) that are related to sarcoidosis:

- **A case of lymphomatoid granulomatosis mimicking sarcoidosis.**
  Author(s): Fitch PS, Smith ME, Davies MG, Prentice AG.
  Source: Respiratory Medicine. 1998 July; 92(7): 966-8. No Abstract Available.
  http://www.ncbi.nlm.nih.gov:80/entrez/query.fcgi?cmd=Retrieve&db=PubMed&list_uids=10070572&dopt=Abstract

- **A perplexing case of hilar adenopathy. Clinical conference in pulmonary disease from the Ohio State University College of Medicine.**
  Author(s): Shaw RA, Schonfeld SA, Whitcomb ME.

Source: Chest. 1981 December; 80(6): 736-40. No Abstract Available.
http://www.ncbi.nlm.nih.gov:80/entrez/query.fcgi?cmd=Retrieve&db=
PubMed&list_uids=7307597&dopt=Abstract

- **A simple spectrophotometric assay of carboxypeptidase N (kininase I) in human serum.**
  Author(s): Schweisfurth H, Reinhart E, Heinrich J, Brugger E.
  Source: J Clin Chem Clin Biochem. 1983 October; 21(10): 605-9.
  http://www.ncbi.nlm.nih.gov:80/entrez/query.fcgi?cmd=Retrieve&db=
  PubMed&list_uids=6644248&dopt=Abstract

- **Acupuncture in general practice.**
  Author(s): Lippman HE.
  Source: J Natl Med Assoc. 1973 January; 65(1): 36-9. No Abstract Available.
  http://www.ncbi.nlm.nih.gov:80/entrez/query.fcgi?cmd=Retrieve&db=
  PubMed&list_uids=4687184&dopt=Abstract

- **Autoimmune thrombocytopenia in sarcoidosis.**
  Author(s): Lawrence HJ, Greenberg BR.
  Source: The American Journal of Medicine. 1985 December; 79(6): 761-4.
  http://www.ncbi.nlm.nih.gov:80/entrez/query.fcgi?cmd=Retrieve&db=
  PubMed&list_uids=4073111&dopt=Abstract

- **Bronchoalveolar lavage. Quantitation of intraalveolar fluid?**
  Author(s): Von Wichert P, Joseph K, Muller B, Franck WM.
  Source: Am Rev Respir Dis. 1993 January; 147(1): 148-52.
  http://www.ncbi.nlm.nih.gov:80/entrez/query.fcgi?cmd=Retrieve&db=
  PubMed&list_uids=8420409&dopt=Abstract

- **Cytotoxic agents for use in dermatology. I.**
  Author(s): McDonald CJ.
  Source: Journal of the American Academy of Dermatology. 1985 May; 12(5 Pt 1): 753-75. Review.
  http://www.ncbi.nlm.nih.gov:80/entrez/query.fcgi?cmd=Retrieve&db=
  PubMed&list_uids=3891799&dopt=Abstract

- **Diffuse pulmonary disease caused by nontuberculous mycobacteria in immunocompetent people (hot tub lung).**
  Author(s): Khoor A, Leslie KO, Tazelaar HD, Helmers RA, Colby TV.

Source: Am J Clin Pathol. 2001 May; 115(5): 755-62.
http://www.ncbi.nlm.nih.gov:80/entrez/query.fcgi?cmd=Retrieve&db=
PubMed&list_uids=11345841&dopt=Abstract

- **Dyspnea self-management in African Americans with chronic lung disease.**
  Author(s): Nield M.
  Source: Heart & Lung : the Journal of Critical Care. 2000 January-
  February; 29(1): 50-5.
  http://www.ncbi.nlm.nih.gov:80/entrez/query.fcgi?cmd=Retrieve&db=
  PubMed&list_uids=10636957&dopt=Abstract

- **Effects of qing-fei-tang (seihai-to) and baicalein, its main component flavonoid, on lucigenin-dependent chemiluminescence and leukotriene B4 synthesis of human alveolar macrophages.**
  Author(s): Tanno Y, Kakuta Y, Aikawa T, Shindoh Y, Ohno I, Takishima T.
  Source: Am J Chin Med. 1988; 16(3-4): 145-54.
  http://www.ncbi.nlm.nih.gov:80/entrez/query.fcgi?cmd=Retrieve&db=
  PubMed&list_uids=2854372&dopt=Abstract

- **Elevation of serum angiotensin-converting-enzyme (ACE) level in sarcoidosis.**
  Author(s): Lieberman J.
  Source: The American Journal of Medicine. 1975 September; 59(3): 365-72.
  http://www.ncbi.nlm.nih.gov:80/entrez/query.fcgi?cmd=Retrieve&db=
  PubMed&list_uids=169692&dopt=Abstract

- **Essentials of physical management and rehabilitation in arthritis.**
  Author(s): Swezey RL.
  Source: Semin Arthritis Rheum. 1974 Summer; 3(4): 349-68. No Abstract
  Available.
  http://www.ncbi.nlm.nih.gov:80/entrez/query.fcgi?cmd=Retrieve&db=
  PubMed&list_uids=4830033&dopt=Abstract

- **Histiocytic lymphoma following resolution of sarcoidosis.**
  Author(s): Foon KA, Filderman A, Gale RP.
  Source: Medical and Pediatric Oncology. 1981; 9(4): 325-31.
  http://www.ncbi.nlm.nih.gov:80/entrez/query.fcgi?cmd=Retrieve&db=
  PubMed&list_uids=7266425&dopt=Abstract

- **Identification of a thermolysin-like metalloendopeptidase in serum: activity in normal subjects and in patients with sarcoidosis.**
  Author(s): Almenoff J, Teirstein AS, Thornton JC, Orlowski M.
  Source: The Journal of Laboratory and Clinical Medicine. 1984 March; 103(3): 420-31.
  http://www.ncbi.nlm.nih.gov:80/entrez/query.fcgi?cmd=Retrieve&db=PubMed&list_uids=6366093&dopt=Abstract

- **Increased angiotensin-converting enzyme in peripheral blood monocytes from patients with sarcoidosis.**
  Author(s): Okabe T, Yamagata K, Fujisawa M, Watanabe J, Takaku F, Lanzillo JJ, Fanburg BL.
  Source: The Journal of Clinical Investigation. 1985 March; 75(3): 911-4.
  http://www.ncbi.nlm.nih.gov:80/entrez/query.fcgi?cmd=Retrieve&db=PubMed&list_uids=2984255&dopt=Abstract

- **Increased intestinal permeability in active pulmonary sarcoidosis.**
  Author(s): Wallaert B, Colombel JF, Adenis A, Marchandise X, Hallgren R, Janin A, Tonnel AB.
  Source: Am Rev Respir Dis. 1992 June; 145(6): 1440-5.
  http://www.ncbi.nlm.nih.gov:80/entrez/query.fcgi?cmd=Retrieve&db=PubMed&list_uids=1596016&dopt=Abstract

- **Life threatening thrombocytopenia in sarcoidosis.**
  Author(s): Larner AJ, Dollery CT, Cox TM, Bloom SR, Scadding JG, Rees AJ.
  Source: Bmj (Clinical Research Ed.). 1990 February 3; 300(6720): 317-9. No Abstract Available.
  http://www.ncbi.nlm.nih.gov:80/entrez/query.fcgi?cmd=Retrieve&db=PubMed&list_uids=2106965&dopt=Abstract

- **Malignant lymphoma of the bone associated with systemic sarcoidosis.**
  Author(s): Kobayashi H, Kato Y, Hakamada M, Hattori Y, Sato A, Shimizu N, Imamura A, Mihara H, Kato H, Oki Y, Morishita M, Miwa H, Nitta M.
  Source: Intern Med. 2001 May; 40(5): 435-8.
  http://www.ncbi.nlm.nih.gov:80/entrez/query.fcgi?cmd=Retrieve&db=PubMed&list_uids=11393419&dopt=Abstract

- **Markedly elevated angiotensin converting enzyme in lymph nodes containing non-necrotizing granulomas in sarcoidosis.**
  Author(s): Silverstein E, Friedland J, Lyons HA, Gourin A.

Source: Proceedings of the National Academy of Sciences of the United States of America. 1976 June; 73(6): 2137-41.
http://www.ncbi.nlm.nih.gov:80/entrez/query.fcgi?cmd=Retrieve&db=PubMed&list_uids=6963&dopt=Abstract

- **No effect of high-dose inhaled steroids in pulmonary sarcoidosis: a double-blind, placebo-controlled study.**
  Author(s): Milman N, Graudal N, Grode G, Munch E.
  Source: Journal of Internal Medicine. 1994 September; 236(3): 285-90.
  http://www.ncbi.nlm.nih.gov:80/entrez/query.fcgi?cmd=Retrieve&db=PubMed&list_uids=8077885&dopt=Abstract

- **Occurrence of sarcoidosis subsequent to chemotherapy for non-Hodgkin's lymphoma: report of two cases.**
  Author(s): Kornacker M, Kraemer A, Leo E, Ho AD.
  Source: Annals of Hematology. 2002 February; 81(2): 103-5.
  http://www.ncbi.nlm.nih.gov:80/entrez/query.fcgi?cmd=Retrieve&db=PubMed&list_uids=11907791&dopt=Abstract

- **Primary care paradigm for management of sarcoidosis, Part 1.**
  Author(s): Young RC Jr, Rachal RE, Nelson-Knuckles B, Arthur CN, Nevels HV.
  Source: J Natl Med Assoc. 1997 March; 89(3): 181-90. Review.
  http://www.ncbi.nlm.nih.gov:80/entrez/query.fcgi?cmd=Retrieve&db=PubMed&list_uids=9094843&dopt=Abstract

- **Primary care paradigm for management of sarcoidosis, Part 2.**
  Author(s): Young RC Jr, Rachal RE, Nelson-Knuckles B, Arthur CN, Nevels HV.
  Source: J Natl Med Assoc. 1997 April; 89(4): 243-52.
  http://www.ncbi.nlm.nih.gov:80/entrez/query.fcgi?cmd=Retrieve&db=PubMed&list_uids=9145629&dopt=Abstract

- **Pulmonary sarcoidosis following interferon therapy for advanced renal cell carcinoma.**
  Author(s): Abdi EA, Nguyen GK, Ludwig RN, Dickout WJ.
  Source: Cancer. 1987 March 1; 59(5): 896-900.
  http://www.ncbi.nlm.nih.gov:80/entrez/query.fcgi?cmd=Retrieve&db=PubMed&list_uids=3815268&dopt=Abstract

- **Sarcoidosis and dermatomyositis in a patient with hemoglobin SC. A case report and literature review.**
  Author(s): Brateanu AC, Caracioni A, Smith HR.
  Source: Sarcoidosis Vasc Diffuse Lung Dis. 2000 June; 17(2): 190-3. Review.
  http://www.ncbi.nlm.nih.gov:80/entrez/query.fcgi?cmd=Retrieve&db=PubMed&list_uids=10957767&dopt=Abstract

- **'Sarcoidosis' and sarcoid-like lesions. Their occurrence after cytotoxic and radiation therapy of testis cancer.**
  Author(s): Trump DL, Ettinger DS, Feldman MJ, Dragon LH.
  Source: Archives of Internal Medicine. 1981 January; 141(1): 37-8. No Abstract Available.
  http://www.ncbi.nlm.nih.gov:80/entrez/query.fcgi?cmd=Retrieve&db=PubMed&list_uids=7447582&dopt=Abstract

- **Sarcoidosis complicated by HTLV III-infection: steroid therapy in combination with thymostimulin.**
  Author(s): Wurm K, Ewert G, Lohr G.
  Source: Sarcoidosis. 1987 March; 4(1): 68-70.
  http://www.ncbi.nlm.nih.gov:80/entrez/query.fcgi?cmd=Retrieve&db=PubMed&list_uids=3589195&dopt=Abstract

- **Sarcoidosis following chemotherapy for Hodgkin's disease.**
  Author(s): Merchant TE, Filippa DA, Yahalom J.
  Source: Leukemia & Lymphoma. 1994 April; 13(3-4): 339-47. Review.
  http://www.ncbi.nlm.nih.gov:80/entrez/query.fcgi?cmd=Retrieve&db=PubMed&list_uids=7519511&dopt=Abstract

- **Sarcoidosis.**
  Author(s): Wright MG.
  Source: The British Journal of Dermatology. 1967 July; 79(7): 421-3. No Abstract Available.
  http://www.ncbi.nlm.nih.gov:80/entrez/query.fcgi?cmd=Retrieve&db=PubMed&list_uids=6029227&dopt=Abstract

- **Sialidase activity and antibodies to sialidase-treated autologous erythrocytes in bronchoalveolar lavages from patients with idiopathic pulmonary fibrosis or sarcoidosis.**
  Author(s): Lambre CR, Pilatte Y, Le Maho S, Greffard A, De Cremoux H, Bignon J.

Source: Clinical and Experimental Immunology. 1988 August; 73(2): 230-5.
http://www.ncbi.nlm.nih.gov:80/entrez/query.fcgi?cmd=Retrieve&db=PubMed&list_uids=3180512&dopt=Abstract

- **Similarity in some properties of serum angiotensin converting enzyme from sarcoidosis patients and normal subjects.**
  Author(s): Friedland J, Silverstein E.
  Source: Biochem Med. 1976 April; 15(2): 178-85. No Abstract Available.
  http://www.ncbi.nlm.nih.gov:80/entrez/query.fcgi?cmd=Retrieve&db=PubMed&list_uids=183757&dopt=Abstract

- **Spontaneous remission or response to methotrexate in sarcoidosis.**
  Author(s): Lacher MJ.
  Source: Annals of Internal Medicine. 1968 December; 69(6): 1247-8. No Abstract Available.
  http://www.ncbi.nlm.nih.gov:80/entrez/query.fcgi?cmd=Retrieve&db=PubMed&list_uids=5725738&dopt=Abstract

Additional Web Resources

A number of additional Web sites offer encyclopedic information covering CAM and related topics. The following is a representative sample:

- Alternative Medicine Foundation, Inc.: **http://www.herbmed.org/**

- AOL: **http://search.aol.com/cat.adp?id=169&layer=&from=subcats**

- Chinese Medicine: **http://www.newcenturynutrition.com/**

- drkoop.com®:
  http://www.drkoop.com/InteractiveMedicine/IndexC.html

- Family Village: **http://www.familyvillage.wisc.edu/med_altn.htm**

- Google: **http://directory.google.com/Top/Health/Alternative/**

- Healthnotes: **http://www.thedacare.org/healthnotes/**

- Open Directory Project: **http://dmoz.org/Health/Alternative/**

- TPN.com: **http://www.tnp.com/**

- Yahoo.com: **http://dir.yahoo.com/Health/Alternative_Medicine/**

- WebMD®Health: **http://my.webmd.com/drugs_and_herbs**

- WellNet: **http://www.wellnet.ca/herbsa-c.htm**

- WholeHealthMD.com:
  http://www.wholehealthmd.com/reflib/0,1529,,00.html

The following is a specific Web list relating to sarcoidosis; please note that any particular subject below may indicate either a therapeutic use, or a contraindication (potential danger), and does not reflect an official recommendation:

- **General Overview**

  Sarcoidosis
  Source: Integrative Medicine Communications; www.onemedicine.com
  Hyperlink:
  http://www.drkoop.com/InteractiveMedicine/ConsLookups/Uses/sar
  coidosis.html

  Sarcoidosis
  Source: Integrative Medicine Communications; www.onemedicine.com
  Hyperlink:
  http://www.drkoop.com/interactivemedicine/ConsConditions/Sarcoid
  osiscc.html

- **Herbs and Supplements**

  Allopurinol
  Source: Integrative Medicine Communications; www.onemedicine.com
  Hyperlink:
  http://www.drkoop.com/interactivemedicine/ConsConditions/Sarcoid
  osiscc.html

  Corticosteroids
  Source: Integrative Medicine Communications; www.onemedicine.com
  Hyperlink:
  http://www.drkoop.com/interactivemedicine/ConsConditions/Sarcoid
  osiscc.html

  Flurbiprofen
  Source: Healthnotes, Inc.; www.healthnotes.com
  Hyperlink:
  http://www.thedacare.org/healthnotes/Drug/Flurbiprofen.htm

Hydroxychloroquine
Source: Healthnotes, Inc.; www.healthnotes.com
Hyperlink:
http://www.thedacare.org/healthnotes/Drug/Hydroxychloroquine.htm

Hydroxychloroquine
Source: Integrative Medicine Communications; www.onemedicine.com
Hyperlink:
http://www.drkoop.com/interactivemedicine/ConsConditions/Sarcoid
osiscc.html

Melatonin
Source: Healthnotes, Inc.; www.healthnotes.com
Hyperlink:
http://www.thedacare.org/healthnotes/Supp/Melatonin.htm

Melatonin
Source: Integrative Medicine Communications; www.onemedicine.com
Hyperlink:
http://www.drkoop.com/interactivemedicine/ConsSupplements/Mela
tonincs.html

Melatonin
Source: Integrative Medicine Communications; www.onemedicine.com
Hyperlink:
http://www.drkoop.com/interactivemedicine/ConsConditions/Sarcoid
osiscc.html

Methotrexate
Source: Integrative Medicine Communications; www.onemedicine.com
Hyperlink:
http://www.drkoop.com/interactivemedicine/ConsConditions/Sarcoid
osiscc.html

Oral Corticosteroids
Source: Integrative Medicine Communications; www.onemedicine.com
Hyperlink:
http://www.drkoop.com/interactivemedicine/ConsConditions/Sarcoid
osiscc.html

Prednisone
Source: Integrative Medicine Communications; www.onemedicine.com

Hyperlink:
http://www.drkoop.com/interactivemedicine/ConsConditions/Sarcoid
osiscc.html

- **Related Conditions**

Hypertension
Alternative names: High Blood Pressure
Source: Prima Communications, Inc.
Hyperlink: http://www.personalhealthzone.com/pg000293.html

Osteoporosis
Source: Prima Communications, Inc.
Hyperlink: http://www.personalhealthzone.com/pg000270.html

PMS
Alternative names: Premenstrual Stress Syndrome
Source: Prima Communications, Inc.
Hyperlink: http://www.personalhealthzone.com/pg000289.html

Uveitis
Source: Integrative Medicine Communications; www.onemedicine.com
Hyperlink:
http://www.drkoop.com/interactivemedicine/ConsConditions/Uveitis
cc.html

General References

A good place to find general background information on CAM is the National Library of Medicine. It has prepared within the MEDLINEplus system an information topic page dedicated to complementary and alternative medicine. To access this page, go to the MEDLINEplus site at: **www.nlm.nih.gov/medlineplus/alternativemedicine.html.** This Web site provides a general overview of various topics and can lead to a number of general sources. The following additional references describe, in broad terms, alternative and complementary medicine (sorted alphabetically by title; hyperlinks provide rankings, information, and reviews at Amazon.com):

- **Alternative Medicine for Dummies** by James Dillard (Author); Audio Cassette, Abridged edition (1998), Harper Audio; ISBN: 0694520659; **http://www.amazon.com/exec/obidos/ASIN/0694520659/icongroupinterna**

- **Complementary and Alternative Medicine Secrets** by W. Kohatsu (Editor); Hardcover (2001), Hanley & Belfus; ISBN: 1560534400; http://www.amazon.com/exec/obidos/ASIN/1560534400/icongroupinterna

- **Dictionary of Alternative Medicine** by J. C. Segen; Paperback-2nd edition (2001), Appleton & Lange; ISBN: 0838516211; http://www.amazon.com/exec/obidos/ASIN/0838516211/icongroupinterna

- **Eat, Drink, and Be Healthy: The Harvard Medical School Guide to Healthy Eating** by Walter C. Willett, MD, et al; Hardcover - 352 pages (2001), Simon & Schuster; ISBN: 0684863375; http://www.amazon.com/exec/obidos/ASIN/0684863375/icongroupinterna

- **Encyclopedia of Natural Medicine, Revised 2nd Edition** by Michael T. Murray, Joseph E. Pizzorno; Paperback - 960 pages, 2nd Rev edition (1997), Prima Publishing; ISBN: 0761511571; http://www.amazon.com/exec/obidos/ASIN/0761511571/icongroupinterna

- **Integrative Medicine: An Introduction to the Art & Science of Healing** by Andrew Weil (Author); Audio Cassette, Unabridged edition (2001), Sounds True; ISBN: 1564558541; http://www.amazon.com/exec/obidos/ASIN/1564558541/icongroupinterna

- **New Encyclopedia of Herbs & Their Uses** by Deni Bown; Hardcover - 448 pages, Revised edition (2001), DK Publishing; ISBN: 078948031X; http://www.amazon.com/exec/obidos/ASIN/078948031X/icongroupinterna

- **Textbook of Complementary and Alternative Medicine** by Wayne B. Jonas; Hardcover (2003), Lippincott, Williams & Wilkins; ISBN: 0683044370; http://www.amazon.com/exec/obidos/ASIN/0683044370/icongroupinterna

For additional information on complementary and alternative medicine, ask your doctor or write to:

National Institutes of Health
National Center for Complementary and Alternative Medicine
Clearinghouse
P. O. Box 8218
Silver Spring, MD 20907-8218

APPENDIX C. RESEARCHING NUTRITION

Overview

Since the time of Hippocrates, doctors have understood the importance of diet and nutrition to patients' health and well-being. Since then, they have accumulated an impressive archive of studies and knowledge dedicated to this subject. Based on their experience, doctors and healthcare providers may recommend particular dietary supplements to patients with sarcoidosis. Any dietary recommendation is based on a patient's age, body mass, gender, lifestyle, eating habits, food preferences, and health condition. It is therefore likely that different patients with sarcoidosis may be given different recommendations. Some recommendations may be directly related to sarcoidosis, while others may be more related to the patient's general health. These recommendations, themselves, may differ from what official sources recommend for the average person.

In this chapter we will begin by briefly reviewing the essentials of diet and nutrition that will broadly frame more detailed discussions of sarcoidosis. We will then show you how to find studies dedicated specifically to nutrition and sarcoidosis.

Food and Nutrition: General Principles

What Are Essential Foods?

Food is generally viewed by official sources as consisting of six basic elements: (1) fluids, (2) carbohydrates, (3) protein, (4) fats, (5) vitamins, and

(6) minerals. Consuming a combination of these elements is considered to be a healthy diet:

- **Fluids** are essential to human life as 80-percent of the body is composed of water. Water is lost via urination, sweating, diarrhea, vomiting, diuretics (drugs that increase urination), caffeine, and physical exertion.

- **Carbohydrates** are the main source for human energy (thermoregulation) and the bulk of typical diets. They are mostly classified as being either simple or complex. Simple carbohydrates include sugars which are often consumed in the form of cookies, candies, or cakes. Complex carbohydrates consist of starches and dietary fibers. Starches are consumed in the form of pastas, breads, potatoes, rice, and other foods. Soluble fibers can be eaten in the form of certain vegetables, fruits, oats, and legumes. Insoluble fibers include brown rice, whole grains, certain fruits, wheat bran and legumes.

- **Proteins** are eaten to build and repair human tissues. Some foods that are high in protein are also high in fat and calories. Food sources for protein include nuts, meat, fish, cheese, and other dairy products.

- **Fats** are consumed for both energy and the absorption of certain vitamins. There are many types of fats, with many general publications recommending the intake of unsaturated fats or those low in cholesterol.

Vitamins and minerals are fundamental to human health, growth, and, in some cases, disease prevention. Most are consumed in your diet (exceptions being vitamins K and D which are produced by intestinal bacteria and sunlight on the skin, respectively). Each vitamin and mineral plays a different role in health. The following outlines essential vitamins:

- **Vitamin A** is important to the health of your eyes, hair, bones, and skin; sources of vitamin A include foods such as eggs, carrots, and cantaloupe.

- **Vitamin B^1**, also known as thiamine, is important for your nervous system and energy production; food sources for thiamine include meat, peas, fortified cereals, bread, and whole grains.

- **Vitamin B^2**, also known as riboflavin, is important for your nervous system and muscles, but is also involved in the release of proteins from nutrients; food sources for riboflavin include dairy products, leafy vegetables, meat, and eggs.

- **Vitamin B^3**, also known as niacin, is important for healthy skin and helps the body use energy; food sources for niacin include peas, peanuts, fish, and whole grains

- **Vitamin B^6**, also known as pyridoxine, is important for the regulation of cells in the nervous system and is vital for blood formation; food sources for pyridoxine include bananas, whole grains, meat, and fish.

- **Vitamin B^{12}** is vital for a healthy nervous system and for the growth of red blood cells in bone marrow; food sources for vitamin B^{12} include yeast, milk, fish, eggs, and meat.

- **Vitamin C** allows the body's immune system to fight various diseases, strengthens body tissue, and improves the body's use of iron; food sources for vitamin C include a wide variety of fruits and vegetables.

- **Vitamin D** helps the body absorb calcium which strengthens bones and teeth; food sources for vitamin D include oily fish and dairy products.

- **Vitamin E** can help protect certain organs and tissues from various degenerative diseases; food sources for vitamin E include margarine, vegetables, eggs, and fish.

- **Vitamin K** is essential for bone formation and blood clotting; common food sources for vitamin K include leafy green vegetables.

- **Folic Acid** maintains healthy cells and blood and, when taken by a pregnant woman, can prevent her fetus from developing neural tube defects; food sources for folic acid include nuts, fortified breads, leafy green vegetables, and whole grains.

It should be noted that one can overdose on certain vitamins which become toxic if consumed in excess (e.g. vitamin A, D, E and K).

Like vitamins, minerals are chemicals that are required by the body to remain in good health. Because the human body does not manufacture these chemicals internally, we obtain them from food and other dietary sources. The more important minerals include:

- **Calcium** is needed for healthy bones, teeth, and muscles, but also helps the nervous system function; food sources for calcium include dry beans, peas, eggs, and dairy products.

- **Chromium** is helpful in regulating sugar levels in blood; food sources for chromium include egg yolks, raw sugar, cheese, nuts, beets, whole grains, and meat.

- **Fluoride** is used by the body to help prevent tooth decay and to reinforce bone strength; sources of fluoride include drinking water and certain brands of toothpaste.

- **Iodine** helps regulate the body's use of energy by synthesizing into the hormone thyroxine; food sources include leafy green vegetables, nuts, egg yolks, and red meat.

- **Iron** helps maintain muscles and the formation of red blood cells and certain proteins; food sources for iron include meat, dairy products, eggs, and leafy green vegetables.

- **Magnesium** is important for the production of DNA, as well as for healthy teeth, bones, muscles, and nerves; food sources for magnesium include dried fruit, dark green vegetables, nuts, and seafood.

- **Phosphorous** is used by the body to work with calcium to form bones and teeth; food sources for phosphorous include eggs, meat, cereals, and dairy products.

- **Selenium** primarily helps maintain normal heart and liver functions; food sources for selenium include wholegrain cereals, fish, meat, and dairy products.

- **Zinc** helps wounds heal, the formation of sperm, and encourage rapid growth and energy; food sources include dried beans, shellfish, eggs, and nuts.

The United States government periodically publishes recommended diets and consumption levels of the various elements of food. Again, your doctor may encourage deviations from the average official recommendation based on your specific condition. To learn more about basic dietary guidelines, visit the Web site: **http://www.health.gov/dietaryguidelines/**. Based on these guidelines, many foods are required to list the nutrition levels on the food's packaging. Labeling Requirements are listed at the following site maintained by the Food and Drug Administration: **http://www.cfsan.fda.gov/~dms/lab-cons.html**. When interpreting these requirements, the government recommends that consumers become familiar with the following abbreviations before reading FDA literature:[50]

- **DVs (Daily Values):** A new dietary reference term that will appear on the food label. It is made up of two sets of references, DRVs and RDIs.

- **DRVs (Daily Reference Values):** A set of dietary references that applies to fat, saturated fat, cholesterol, carbohydrate, protein, fiber, sodium, and potassium.

- **RDIs (Reference Daily Intakes):** A set of dietary references based on the Recommended Dietary Allowances for essential vitamins and minerals

---

[50] Adapted from the FDA: **http://www.fda.gov/fdac/special/foodlabel/dvs.html**.

and, in selected groups, protein. The name "RDI" replaces the term "U.S. RDA."

- **RDAs (Recommended Dietary Allowances):** A set of estimated nutrient allowances established by the National Academy of Sciences. It is updated periodically to reflect current scientific knowledge.

What Are Dietary Supplements?[51]

Dietary supplements are widely available through many commercial sources, including health food stores, grocery stores, pharmacies, and by mail. Dietary supplements are provided in many forms including tablets, capsules, powders, gel-tabs, extracts, and liquids. Historically in the United States, the most prevalent type of dietary supplement was a multivitamin/mineral tablet or capsule that was available in pharmacies, either by prescription or "over the counter." Supplements containing strictly herbal preparations were less widely available. Currently in the United States, a wide array of supplement products are available, including vitamin, mineral, other nutrients, and botanical supplements as well as ingredients and extracts of animal and plant origin.

The Office of Dietary Supplements (ODS) of the National Institutes of Health is the official agency of the United States which has the expressed goal of acquiring "new knowledge to help prevent, detect, diagnose, and treat disease and disability, from the rarest genetic disorder to the common cold."[52] According to the ODS, dietary supplements can have an important impact on the prevention and management of disease and on the maintenance of health.[53] The ODS notes that considerable research on the effects of dietary supplements has been conducted in Asia and Europe where the use of plant products, in particular, has a long tradition. However, the overwhelming majority of supplements have not been studied scientifically.

---

[51] This discussion has been adapted from the NIH:
http://ods.od.nih.gov/whatare/whatare.html.

[52] Contact: The Office of Dietary Supplements, National Institutes of Health, Building 31, Room 1B29, 31 Center Drive, MSC 2086, Bethesda, Maryland 20892-2086, Tel: (301) 435-2920, Fax: (301) 480-1845, E-mail: **ods@nih.gov**.

[53] Adapted from **http://ods.od.nih.gov/about/about.html**. The Dietary Supplement Health and Education Act defines dietary supplements as "a product (other than tobacco) intended to supplement the diet that bears or contains one or more of the following dietary ingredients: a vitamin, mineral, amino acid, herb or other botanical; or a dietary substance for use to supplement the diet by increasing the total dietary intake; or a concentrate, metabolite, constituent, extract, or combination of any ingredient described above; and intended for ingestion in the form of a capsule, powder, softgel, or gelcap, and not represented as a conventional food or as a sole item of a meal or the diet."

To explore the role of dietary supplements in the improvement of health care, the ODS plans, organizes, and supports conferences, workshops, and symposia on scientific topics related to dietary supplements. The ODS often works in conjunction with other NIH Institutes and Centers, other government agencies, professional organizations, and public advocacy groups.

To learn more about official information on dietary supplements, visit the ODS site at **http://ods.od.nih.gov/whatare/whatare.html**. Or contact:

> The Office of Dietary Supplements
> National Institutes of Health
> Building 31, Room 1B29
> 31 Center Drive, MSC 2086
> Bethesda, Maryland 20892-2086
> Tel: (301) 435-2920
> Fax: (301) 480-1845
> E-mail: ods@nih.gov

Finding Studies on Sarcoidosis

The NIH maintains an office dedicated to patient nutrition and diet. The National Institutes of Health's Office of Dietary Supplements (ODS) offers a searchable bibliographic database called the IBIDS (International Bibliographic Information on Dietary Supplements). The IBIDS contains over 460,000 scientific citations and summaries about dietary supplements and nutrition as well as references to published international, scientific literature on dietary supplements such as vitamins, minerals, and botanicals.[54] IBIDS is available to the public free of charge through the ODS Internet page: **http://ods.od.nih.gov/databases/ibids.html**.

After entering the search area, you have three choices: (1) IBIDS Consumer Database, (2) Full IBIDS Database, or (3) Peer Reviewed Citations Only. We recommend that you start with the Consumer Database. While you may not find references for the topics that are of most interest to you, check back periodically as this database is frequently updated. More studies can be

---

[54] Adapted from http://ods.od.nih.gov. IBIDS is produced by the Office of Dietary Supplements (ODS) at the National Institutes of Health to assist the public, healthcare providers, educators, and researchers in locating credible, scientific information on dietary supplements. IBIDS was developed and will be maintained through an interagency partnership with the Food and Nutrition Information Center of the National Agricultural Library, U.S. Department of Agriculture.

found by searching the Full IBIDS Database. Healthcare professionals and researchers generally use the third option, which lists peer-reviewed citations. In all cases, we suggest that you take advantage of the "Advanced Search" option that allows you to retrieve up to 100 fully explained references in a comprehensive format. Type "sarcoidosis" (or synonyms) into the search box. To narrow the search, you can also select the "Title" field.

The following information is typical of that found when using the "Full IBIDS Database" when searching using "sarcoidosis" (or a synonym):

- **A case of sarcoidosis involving the tongue.**
  Author(s): Department of Dermatology, Kagoshima University Faculty of Medicine, Japan.
  Source: Nagata, Y Kanekura, T Kawabata, H Shimomai, K Higashi, Y Setoyama, M Kanzaki, T J-Dermatol. 1999 October; 26(10): 666-70 0385-2407

- **Acne fulminans and erythema nodosum during isotretinoin therapy responding to dapsone.**
  Author(s): Department of Dermatology, Central Outpatients, Stoke-on-Trent, UK.
  Source: Tan, B B Lear, J T Smith, A G Clin-Exp-Dermatol. 1997 January; 22(1): 26-7 0307-6938

- **Antemortem diagnosis of cardiac sarcoidosis by abnormal uptake of 201Tl in bilateral hilar lymph nodes.**
  Author(s): Second Department of Medicine, Kyoto Prefectural University of Medicine, Japan.
  Source: Nakamura, T Sugihara, H Narihara, R Adachi, H Nakagawa, M Ann-Nucl-Med. 1994 November; 8(4): 295-8 0914-7187

- **Beryllium workers--sarcoidosis or chronic beryllium disease.**
  Author(s): Histopathology Department, University of Wales College of Medicine, Llandough Hospital, South Glamorgan, Great Britain.
  Source: Williams, W J Sarcoidosis. 1989 October; 6 Suppl 134-5 0393-1447

- **Biochemical changes in sarcoidosis.**
  Author(s): Department of Pneumology and Allergology, Ruhrlandklinik, Essen, Germany.
  Source: Costabel, U Teschler, H Clin-Chest-Med. 1997 December; 18(4): 827-42 0272-5231

- **Bone protection with salmon calcitonin (sCT) in the long-term steroid therapy of chronic sarcoidosis.**
  Author(s): Sarcoidosis Clinic, Niguarda Hospital, Milan, Italy.

Source: Rizzato, G Tosi, G Schiraldi, G Montemurro, L Zanni, D Sisti, S Sarcoidosis. 1988 September; 5(2): 99-103 0393-1447

- **Bone sarcoidosis.**
  Author(s): LAC+USC Medical Center, Los Angeles, California 90033, USA.
  Source: Wilcox, A Bharadwaj, P Sharma, O P Curr-Opin-Rheumatol. 2000 July; 12(4): 321-30 1040-8711

- **Calcium oxalate and iron accumulation in sarcoidosis.**
  Author(s): Department of Medicine, Duke University Medical Center, Durham, NC 27710, USA.
  Source: Ghio, A J Roggli, V L Kennedy, T P Piantadosi, C A Sarcoidosis-Vasc-Diffuse-Lung-Dis. 2000 June; 17(2): 140-50 1124-0490

- **Chlorambucil treatment of sarcoidosis.**
  Author(s): Department of Medicine, Jefferson Medical College, Philadelphia, PA 19107.
  Source: Israel, H L McComb, B L Sarcoidosis. 1991 March; 8(1): 35-41 0393-1447

- **Confluent choroidal infiltrates with sarcoidosis.**
  Author(s): Department of Ophthalmology, Mayo Clinic, Rochester, Minnesota 55905, USA.
  Source: Cook, B E Robertson, D M Retina. 2000; 20(1): 1-7 0275-004X

- **Corticosteroid therapy in sarcoidosis. A five-year, controlled follow-up study.**
  Source: Zaki, M H Lyons, H A Leilop, L Huang, C T N-Y-State-J-Med. 1987 September; 87(9): 496-9 0028-7628

- **Corticosteroid treatment of sarcoidosis--who needs it?**
  Source: Israel, H L N-Y-State-J-Med. 1987 September; 87(9): 490 0028-7628

- **Corticosteroids for pulmonary sarcoidosis.**
  Author(s): Division of Physiological Medicine, St George's Hospital Medical School, Cranmer Terrace, London, UK, SW17 0RE.
  Source: Paramothayan, N S Jones, P W Cochrane-Database-Syst-Revolume 2000; (2): CD001114 1469-493X

- **Diagnosis, pathogenesis, and treatment of sarcoidosis.**
  Author(s): Division of Pulmonary and Critical Care Medicine, University of Southern California School of Medicine, Los Angeles 90033, USA.
  Source: Sharma, O P Alam, S Curr-Opin-Pulm-Med. 1995 September; 1(5): 392-400 1078-1641

- **Differential response to corticosteroid therapy of MRI findings and clinical manifestations in spinal cord sarcoidosis.**
  Author(s): Department of Neurology, Nagoya University School of Medicine, Japan.
  Source: Koike, H Misu, K Yasui, K Kameyama, T Ando, T Yanagi, T Sobue, G J-Neurol. 2000 July; 247(7): 544-9 0340-5354

- **Elevated serum levels of soluble interleukin-2 receptors in active pulmonary sarcoidosis: relative specificity and association with hypercalcemia.**
  Author(s): Rockwell-Keough Pulmonary Immunology Laboratory, Methodist Hospital, Houston, Texas 77030.
  Source: Lawrence, E C Berger, M B Brousseau, K P Rodriguez, T M Siegel, S J Kurman, C C Nelson, D L Sarcoidosis. 1987 September; 4(2): 87-93 0393-1447

- **Endocrine complications of sarcoidosis.**
  Author(s): Veterans Affairs Medical Center, Charleston, South Carolina.
  Source: Bell, N H Endocrinol-Metab-Clin-North-Am. 1991 September; 20(3): 645-54 0889-8529

- **Enhanced cell-mediated immune responses in erythema nodosum leprosum reactions of leprosy.**
  Source: Rao, T D Rao, P R Int-J-Lepr-Other-Mycobact-Dis. 1987 March; 55(1): 36-41 0148-916X

- **Erythema nodosum and non-Hodgkin's lymphoma.**
  Author(s): Section of Rheumatology, Wellesley Hospital, Toronto, Canada.
  Source: Thomson, G T Keystone, E C Sturgeon, J F Fornasier, V J-Rheumatol. 1990 March; 17(3): 383-5 0315-162X

- **Erythema nodosum associated with acute cytomegalovirus mononucleosis in an adult.**
  Author(s): Department of Medicine, Rush-Presbyterian-St Luke's Medical Center, Chicago.
  Source: Spear, J B Kessler, H A Dworin, A Semel, J Arch-Intern-Med. 1988 February; 148(2): 323-4 0003-9926

Federal Resources on Nutrition

In addition to the IBIDS, the United States Department of Health and Human Services (HHS) and the United States Department of Agriculture (USDA) provide many sources of information on general nutrition and health. Recommended resources include:

- healthfinder®, HHS's gateway to health information, including diet and nutrition:
  http://www.healthfinder.gov/scripts/SearchContext.asp?topic=238&page=0

- The United States Department of Agriculture's Web site dedicated to nutrition information: **www.nutrition.gov**

- The Food and Drug Administration's Web site for federal food safety information: **www.foodsafety.gov**

- The National Action Plan on Overweight and Obesity sponsored by the United States Surgeon General:
  http://www.surgeongeneral.gov/topics/obesity/

- The Center for Food Safety and Applied Nutrition has an Internet site sponsored by the Food and Drug Administration and the Department of Health and Human Services: **http://vm.cfsan.fda.gov/**

- Center for Nutrition Policy and Promotion sponsored by the United States Department of Agriculture: **http://www.usda.gov/cnpp/**

- Food and Nutrition Information Center, National Agricultural Library sponsored by the United States Department of Agriculture: **http://www.nal.usda.gov/fnic/**

- Food and Nutrition Service sponsored by the United States Department of Agriculture: **http://www.fns.usda.gov/fns/**

Additional Web Resources

A number of additional Web sites offer encyclopedic information covering food and nutrition. The following is a representative sample:

- AOL: **http://search.aol.com/cat.adp?id=174&layer=&from=subcats**

- Family Village: **http://www.familyvillage.wisc.edu/med_nutrition.html**

- Google: **http://directory.google.com/Top/Health/Nutrition/**

- Healthnotes: **http://www.thedacare.org/healthnotes/**

- Open Directory Project: **http://dmoz.org/Health/Nutrition/**

- Yahoo.com: **http://dir.yahoo.com/Health/Nutrition/**

- WebMD®Health: **http://my.webmd.com/nutrition**

- WholeHealthMD.com:
  http://www.wholehealthmd.com/reflib/0,1529,,00.html

The following is a specific Web list relating to sarcoidosis; please note that any particular subject below may indicate either a therapeutic use, or a contraindication (potential danger), and does not reflect an official recommendation:

- **Vitamins**

  Vitamin D
  Source: Healthnotes, Inc.; www.healthnotes.com
  Hyperlink:
  http://www.thedacare.org/healthnotes/Supp/Vitamin_D.htm

  Vitamin D
  Source: Prima Communications, Inc.
  Hyperlink: http://www.personalhealthzone.com/pg000129.html

- **Minerals**

  Calcium
  Source: Integrative Medicine Communications; www.onemedicine.com
  Hyperlink:
  http://www.drkoop.com/interactivemedicine/ConsConditions/Sarcoid osiscc.html

  Calcium
  Source: Prima Communications, Inc.
  Hyperlink: http://www.personalhealthzone.com/pg000113.html

  Isotretinoin
  Source: Integrative Medicine Communications; www.onemedicine.com
  Hyperlink:
  http://www.drkoop.com/interactivemedicine/ConsConditions/Sarcoid osiscc.html

- **Food and Diet**

   Diabetes
   Source: Integrative Medicine Communications; www.onemedicine.com
   Hyperlink:
   http://www.drkoop.com/interactivemedicine/ConsConditions/Sarcoid
   osiscc.html

Vocabulary Builder

The following vocabulary builder defines words used in the references in this chapter that have not been defined in previous chapters:

Calcitonin: A peptide hormone that lowers calcium concentration in the blood. In humans, it is released by thyroid cells and acts to decrease the formation and absorptive activity of osteoclasts. Its role in regulating plasma calcium is much greater in children and in certain diseases than in normal adults. [NIH]

Carbohydrates: A nutrient that supplies 4 calories/gram. They may be simple or complex. Simple carbohydrates are called sugars, and complex carbohydrates are called starch and fiber (cellulose). An organic compound—containing carbon, hydrogen, and oxygen—that is formed by photosynthesis in plants. Carbohydrates are heat producing and are classified as monosaccharides, disaccharides, or polysaccharides. [NIH]

Cholesterol: A soft, waxy substance manufactured by the body and used in the production of hormones, bile acid, and vitamin D and present in all parts of the body, including the nervous system, muscle, skin, liver, intestines, and heart. Blood cholesterol circulates in the bloodstream. Dietary cholesterol is found in foods of animal origin. [NIH]

Degenerative: Undergoing degeneration : tending to degenerate; having the character of or involving degeneration; causing or tending to cause degeneration. [EU]

Fetus: Unborn offspring from 7 or 8 weeks after conception until birth. [NIH]

Iodine: A nonmetallic element of the halogen group that is represented by the atomic symbol I, atomic number 53, and atomic weight of 126.90. It is a nutritionally essential element, especially important in thyroid hormone synthesis. In solution, it has anti-infective properties and is used topically. [NIH]

Isotretinoin: A topical dermatologic agent that is used in the treatment of acne vulgaris and several other skin diseases. The drug has teratogenic and other adverse effects. [NIH]

Leprosy: A chronic granulomatous infection caused by mycobacterium leprae. The granulomatous lesions are manifested in the skin, the mucous membranes, and the peripheral nerves. Two polar or principal types are lepromatous and tuberculoid. [NIH]

Mononucleosis: The presence of an abnormally large number of mononuclear leucocytes (monocytes) in the blood. The term is often used alone to refer to infectious mononucleosis. [EU]

Neurology: A medical specialty concerned with the study of the structures, functions, and diseases of the nervous system. [NIH]

Niacin: Water-soluble vitamin of the B complex occurring in various animal and plant tissues. Required by the body for the formation of coenzymes NAD and NADP. Has pellagra-curative, vasodilating, and antilipemic properties. [NIH]

Outpatients: Persons who receive ambulatory care at an outpatient department or clinic without room and board being provided. [NIH]

Overweight: An excess of body weight but not necessarily body fat; a body mass index of 25 to 29.9 kg/m2. [NIH]

Selenium: An element with the atomic symbol Se, atomic number 34, and atomic weight 78.96. It is an essential micronutrient for mammals and other animals but is toxic in large amounts. Selenium protects intracellular structures against oxidative damage. It is an essential component of glutathione peroxidase. [NIH]

Thyroxine: An amino acid of the thyroid gland which exerts a stimulating effect on thyroid metabolism. [NIH]

APPENDIX D. FINDING MEDICAL LIBRARIES

Overview

At a medical library you can find medical texts and reference books, consumer health publications, specialty newspapers and magazines, as well as medical journals. In this Appendix, we show you how to quickly find a medical library in your area.

Preparation

Before going to the library, highlight the references mentioned in this sourcebook that you find interesting. Focus on those items that are not available via the Internet, and ask the reference librarian for help with your search. He or she may know of additional resources that could be helpful to you. Most importantly, your local public library and medical libraries have Interlibrary Loan programs with the National Library of Medicine (NLM), one of the largest medical collections in the world. According to the NLM, most of the literature in the general and historical collections of the National Library of Medicine is available on interlibrary loan to any library. NLM's interlibrary loan services are only available to libraries. If you would like to access NLM medical literature, then visit a library in your area that can request the publications for you.[55]

---

[55] Adapted from the NLM: http://www.nlm.nih.gov/psd/cas/interlibrary.html.

Finding a Local Medical Library

The quickest method to locate medical libraries is to use the Internet-based directory published by the National Network of Libraries of Medicine (NN/LM). This network includes 4626 members and affiliates that provide many services to librarians, health professionals, and the public. To find a library in your area, simply visit **http://nnlm.gov/members/adv.html** or call 1-800-338-7657.

Medical Libraries Open to the Public

In addition to the NN/LM, the National Library of Medicine (NLM) lists a number of libraries that are generally open to the public and have reference facilities. The following is the NLM's list plus hyperlinks to each library Web site. These Web pages can provide information on hours of operation and other restrictions. The list below is a small sample of libraries recommended by the National Library of Medicine (sorted alphabetically by name of the U.S. state or Canadian province where the library is located):[56]

- **Alabama:** Health InfoNet of Jefferson County (Jefferson County Library Cooperative, Lister Hill Library of the Health Sciences), **http://www.uab.edu/infonet/**

- **Alabama:** Richard M. Scrushy Library (American Sports Medicine Institute), **http://www.asmi.org/LIBRARY.HTM**

- **Arizona:** Samaritan Regional Medical Center: The Learning Center (Samaritan Health System, Phoenix, Arizona), **http://www.samaritan.edu/library/bannerlibs.htm**

- **California:** Kris Kelly Health Information Center (St. Joseph Health System), **http://www.humboldt1.com/~kkhic/index.html**

- **California:** Community Health Library of Los Gatos (Community Health Library of Los Gatos), **http://www.healthlib.org/orgresources.html**

- **California:** Consumer Health Program and Services (CHIPS) (County of Los Angeles Public Library, Los Angeles County Harbor-UCLA Medical Center Library) - Carson, CA, **http://www.colapublib.org/services/chips.html**

- **California:** Gateway Health Library (Sutter Gould Medical Foundation)

- **California:** Health Library (Stanford University Medical Center), **http://www-med.stanford.edu/healthlibrary/**

- **California:** Patient Education Resource Center - Health Information and Resources (University of California, San Francisco), **http://sfghdean.ucsf.edu/barnett/PERC/default.asp**

- **California:** Redwood Health Library (Petaluma Health Care District), **http://www.phcd.org/rdwdlib.html**

- **California:** San José PlaneTree Health Library, **http://planetreesanjose.org/**

- **California:** Sutter Resource Library (Sutter Hospitals Foundation), **http://go.sutterhealth.org/comm/resc-library/sac-resources.html**

- **California:** University of California, Davis. Health Sciences Libraries

- **California:** ValleyCare Health Library & Ryan Comer Cancer Resource Center (ValleyCare Health System), **http://www.valleycare.com/library.html**

- **California:** Washington Community Health Resource Library (Washington Community Health Resource Library), **http://www.healthlibrary.org/**

- **Colorado:** William V. Gervasini Memorial Library (Exempla Healthcare), **http://www.exempla.org/conslib.htm**

- **Connecticut:** Hartford Hospital Health Science Libraries (Hartford Hospital), **http://www.harthosp.org/library/**

- **Connecticut:** Healthnet: Connecticut Consumer Health Information Center (University of Connecticut Health Center, Lyman Maynard Stowe Library), **http://library.uchc.edu/departm/hnet/**

- **Connecticut:** Waterbury Hospital Health Center Library (Waterbury Hospital), **http://www.waterburyhospital.com/library/consumer.shtml**

- **Delaware:** Consumer Health Library (Christiana Care Health System, Eugene du Pont Preventive Medicine & Rehabilitation Institute), **http://www.christianacare.org/health_guide/health_guide_pmri_health _info.cfm**

- **Delaware:** Lewis B. Flinn Library (Delaware Academy of Medicine), **http://www.delamed.org/chls.html**

- **Georgia:** Family Resource Library (Medical College of Georgia), **http://cmc.mcg.edu/kids_families/fam_resources/fam_res_lib/frl.htm**

- **Georgia:** Health Resource Center (Medical Center of Central Georgia), **http://www.mccg.org/hrc/hrchome.asp**

- **Hawaii:** Hawaii Medical Library: Consumer Health Information Service (Hawaii Medical Library), **http://hml.org/CHIS/**

- **Idaho:** DeArmond Consumer Health Library (Kootenai Medical Center), **http://www.nicon.org/DeArmond/index.htm**

- **Illinois:** Health Learning Center of Northwestern Memorial Hospital (Northwestern Memorial Hospital, Health Learning Center), **http://www.nmh.org/health_info/hlc.html**

- **Illinois:** Medical Library (OSF Saint Francis Medical Center), **http://www.osfsaintfrancis.org/general/library/**

- **Kentucky:** Medical Library - Services for Patients, Families, Students & the Public (Central Baptist Hospital), **http://www.centralbap.com/education/community/library.htm**

- **Kentucky:** University of Kentucky - Health Information Library (University of Kentucky, Chandler Medical Center, Health Information Library), **http://www.mc.uky.edu/PatientEd/**

- **Louisiana:** Alton Ochsner Medical Foundation Library (Alton Ochsner Medical Foundation), **http://www.ochsner.org/library/**

- **Louisiana:** Louisiana State University Health Sciences Center Medical Library-Shreveport, **http://lib-sh.lsuhsc.edu/**

- **Maine:** Franklin Memorial Hospital Medical Library (Franklin Memorial Hospital), **http://www.fchn.org/fmh/lib.htm**

- **Maine:** Gerrish-True Health Sciences Library (Central Maine Medical Center), **http://www.cmmc.org/library/library.html**

- **Maine:** Hadley Parrot Health Science Library (Eastern Maine Healthcare), **http://www.emh.org/hll/hpl/guide.htm**

- **Maine:** Maine Medical Center Library (Maine Medical Center), **http://www.mmc.org/library/**

- **Maine:** Parkview Hospital, **http://www.parkviewhospital.org/communit.htm#Library**

- **Maine:** Southern Maine Medical Center Health Sciences Library (Southern Maine Medical Center), **http://www.smmc.org/services/service.php3?choice=10**

- **Maine:** Stephens Memorial Hospital Health Information Library (Western Maine Health), **http://www.wmhcc.com/hil_frame.html**

- **Manitoba, Canada:** Consumer & Patient Health Information Service (University of Manitoba Libraries), **http://www.umanitoba.ca/libraries/units/health/reference/chis.html**

- **Manitoba, Canada:** J.W. Crane Memorial Library (Deer Lodge Centre), **http://www.deerlodge.mb.ca/library/libraryservices.shtml**

- **Maryland:** Health Information Center at the Wheaton Regional Library (Montgomery County, Md., Dept. of Public Libraries, Wheaton Regional Library), **http://www.mont.lib.md.us/healthinfo/hic.asp**

- **Massachusetts:** Baystate Medical Center Library (Baystate Health System), **http://www.baystatehealth.com/1024/**

- **Massachusetts:** Boston University Medical Center Alumni Medical Library (Boston University Medical Center), **http://med-libwww.bu.edu/library/lib.html**

- **Massachusetts:** Lowell General Hospital Health Sciences Library (Lowell General Hospital), **http://www.lowellgeneral.org/library/HomePageLinks/WWW.htm**

- **Massachusetts:** Paul E. Woodard Health Sciences Library (New England Baptist Hospital), **http://www.nebh.org/health_lib.asp**

- **Massachusetts:** St. Luke's Hospital Health Sciences Library (St. Luke's Hospital), **http://www.southcoast.org/library/**

- **Massachusetts:** Treadwell Library Consumer Health Reference Center (Massachusetts General Hospital), **http://www.mgh.harvard.edu/library/chrcindex.html**

- **Massachusetts:** UMass HealthNet (University of Massachusetts Medical School), **http://healthnet.umassmed.edu/**

- **Michigan:** Botsford General Hospital Library - Consumer Health (Botsford General Hospital, Library & Internet Services), **http://www.botsfordlibrary.org/consumer.htm**

- **Michigan:** Helen DeRoy Medical Library (Providence Hospital and Medical Centers), **http://www.providence-hospital.org/library/**

- **Michigan:** Marquette General Hospital - Consumer Health Library (Marquette General Hospital, Health Information Center), **http://www.mgh.org/center.html**

- **Michigan:** Patient Education Resouce Center - University of Michigan Cancer Center (University of Michigan Comprehensive Cancer Center), **http://www.cancer.med.umich.edu/learn/leares.htm**

- **Michigan:** Sladen Library & Center for Health Information Resources - Consumer Health Information, **http://www.sladen.hfhs.org/library/consumer/index.html**

- **Montana:** Center for Health Information (St. Patrick Hospital and Health Sciences Center), **http://www.saintpatrick.org/chi/librarydetail.php3?ID=41**

- **National:** Consumer Health Library Directory (Medical Library Association, Consumer and Patient Health Information Section), **http://caphis.mlanet.org/directory/index.html**

- **National:** National Network of Libraries of Medicine (National Library of Medicine) - provides library services for health professionals in the United States who do not have access to a medical library, **http://nnlm.gov/**

- **National:** NN/LM List of Libraries Serving the Public (National Network of Libraries of Medicine), **http://nnlm.gov/members/**

- **Nevada:** Health Science Library, West Charleston Library (Las Vegas Clark County Library District), **http://www.lvccld.org/special_collections/medical/index.htm**

- **New Hampshire:** Dartmouth Biomedical Libraries (Dartmouth College Library), **http://www.dartmouth.edu/~biomed/resources.htmld/conshealth.htmld/**

- **New Jersey:** Consumer Health Library (Rahway Hospital), **http://www.rahwayhospital.com/library.htm**

- **New Jersey:** Dr. Walter Phillips Health Sciences Library (Englewood Hospital and Medical Center), **http://www.englewoodhospital.com/links/index.htm**

- **New Jersey:** Meland Foundation (Englewood Hospital and Medical Center), **http://www.geocities.com/ResearchTriangle/9360/**

- **New York:** Choices in Health Information (New York Public Library) - NLM Consumer Pilot Project participant, **http://www.nypl.org/branch/health/links.html**

- **New York:** Health Information Center (Upstate Medical University, State University of New York), **http://www.upstate.edu/library/hic/**

- **New York:** Health Sciences Library (Long Island Jewish Medical Center), **http://www.lij.edu/library/library.html**

- **New York:** ViaHealth Medical Library (Rochester General Hospital), **http://www.nyam.org/library/**

- **Ohio:** Consumer Health Library (Akron General Medical Center, Medical & Consumer Health Library), **http://www.akrongeneral.org/hwlibrary.htm**

- **Oklahoma:** Saint Francis Health System Patient/Family Resource Center (Saint Francis Health System), **http://www.sfh-tulsa.com/patientfamilycenter/default.asp**

- **Oregon:** Planetree Health Resource Center (Mid-Columbia Medical Center), **http://www.mcmc.net/phrc/**

- **Pennsylvania:** Community Health Information Library (Milton S. Hershey Medical Center), **http://www.hmc.psu.edu/commhealth/**

- **Pennsylvania:** Community Health Resource Library (Geisinger Medical Center), **http://www.geisinger.edu/education/commlib.shtml**

- **Pennsylvania:** HealthInfo Library (Moses Taylor Hospital), **http://www.mth.org/healthwellness.html**

- **Pennsylvania:** Hopwood Library (University of Pittsburgh, Health Sciences Library System), **http://www.hsls.pitt.edu/chi/hhrcinfo.html**

- **Pennsylvania:** Koop Community Health Information Center (College of Physicians of Philadelphia), **http://www.collphyphil.org/kooppg1.shtml**

- **Pennsylvania:** Learning Resources Center - Medical Library (Susquehanna Health System), **http://www.shscares.org/services/lrc/index.asp**

- **Pennsylvania:** Medical Library (UPMC Health System), **http://www.upmc.edu/passavant/library.htm**

- **Quebec, Canada:** Medical Library (Montreal General Hospital), **http://ww2.mcgill.ca/mghlib/**

- **South Dakota:** Rapid City Regional Hospital - Health Information Center (Rapid City Regional Hospital, Health Information Center), **http://www.rcrh.org/education/LibraryResourcesConsumers.htm**

- **Texas:** Houston HealthWays (Houston Academy of Medicine-Texas Medical Center Library), **http://hhw.library.tmc.edu/**

- **Texas:** Matustik Family Resource Center (Cook Children's Health Care System), **http://www.cookchildrens.com/Matustik_Library.html**

- **Washington:** Community Health Library (Kittitas Valley Community Hospital), **http://www.kvch.com/**

- **Washington:** Southwest Washington Medical Center Library (Southwest Washington Medical Center), **http://www.swmedctr.com/Home/**

APPENDIX E. YOUR RIGHTS AND INSURANCE

Overview

Any patient with sarcoidosis faces a series of issues related more to the healthcare industry than to the medical condition itself. This appendix covers two important topics in this regard: your rights and responsibilities as a patient, and how to get the most out of your medical insurance plan.

Your Rights as a Patient

The President's Advisory Commission on Consumer Protection and Quality in the Healthcare Industry has created the following summary of your rights as a patient.[57]

Information Disclosure

Consumers have the right to receive accurate, easily understood information. Some consumers require assistance in making informed decisions about health plans, health professionals, and healthcare facilities. Such information includes:

- *Health plans.* Covered benefits, cost-sharing, and procedures for resolving complaints, licensure, certification, and accreditation status, comparable measures of quality and consumer satisfaction, provider

---

[57] Adapted from Consumer Bill of Rights and Responsibilities:
http://www.hcqualitycommission.gov/press/cbor.html#head1.

network composition, the procedures that govern access to specialists and emergency services, and care management information.

- *Health professionals.* Education, board certification, and recertification, years of practice, experience performing certain procedures, and comparable measures of quality and consumer satisfaction.

- *Healthcare facilities.* Experience in performing certain procedures and services, accreditation status, comparable measures of quality, worker, and consumer satisfaction, and procedures for resolving complaints.

- *Consumer assistance programs.* Programs must be carefully structured to promote consumer confidence and to work cooperatively with health plans, providers, payers, and regulators. Desirable characteristics of such programs are sponsorship that ensures accountability to the interests of consumers and stable, adequate funding.

Choice of Providers and Plans

Consumers have the right to a choice of healthcare providers that is sufficient to ensure access to appropriate high-quality healthcare. To ensure such choice, the Commission recommends the following:

- *Provider network adequacy.* All health plan networks should provide access to sufficient numbers and types of providers to assure that all covered services will be accessible without unreasonable delay -- including access to emergency services 24 hours a day and 7 days a week. If a health plan has an insufficient number or type of providers to provide a covered benefit with the appropriate degree of specialization, the plan should ensure that the consumer obtains the benefit outside the network at no greater cost than if the benefit were obtained from participating providers.

- *Women's health services.* Women should be able to choose a qualified provider offered by a plan -- such as gynecologists, certified nurse midwives, and other qualified healthcare providers -- for the provision of covered care necessary to provide routine and preventative women's healthcare services.

- *Access to specialists.* Consumers with complex or serious medical conditions who require frequent specialty care should have direct access to a qualified specialist of their choice within a plan's network of providers. Authorizations, when required, should be for an adequate number of direct access visits under an approved treatment plan.

- *Transitional care.* Consumers who are undergoing a course of treatment for a chronic or disabling condition (or who are in the second or third trimester of a pregnancy) at the time they involuntarily change health plans or at a time when a provider is terminated by a plan for other than cause should be able to continue seeing their current specialty providers for up to 90 days (or through completion of postpartum care) to allow for transition of care.

- *Choice of health plans.* Public and private group purchasers should, wherever feasible, offer consumers a choice of high-quality health insurance plans.

Access to Emergency Services

Consumers have the right to access emergency healthcare services when and where the need arises. Health plans should provide payment when a consumer presents to an emergency department with acute symptoms of sufficient severity--including severe pain--such that a "prudent layperson" could reasonably expect the absence of medical attention to result in placing that consumer's health in serious jeopardy, serious impairment to bodily functions, or serious dysfunction of any bodily organ or part.

Participation in Treatment Decisions

Consumers have the right and responsibility to fully participate in all decisions related to their healthcare. Consumers who are unable to fully participate in treatment decisions have the right to be represented by parents, guardians, family members, or other conservators. Physicians and other health professionals should:

- Provide patients with sufficient information and opportunity to decide among treatment options consistent with the informed consent process.

- Discuss all treatment options with a patient in a culturally competent manner, including the option of no treatment at all.

- Ensure that persons with disabilities have effective communications with members of the health system in making such decisions.

- Discuss all current treatments a consumer may be undergoing.

- Discuss all risks, benefits, and consequences to treatment or nontreatment.

- Give patients the opportunity to refuse treatment and to express preferences about future treatment decisions.

- Discuss the use of advance directives -- both living wills and durable powers of attorney for healthcare -- with patients and their designated family members.

- Abide by the decisions made by their patients and/or their designated representatives consistent with the informed consent process.

Health plans, health providers, and healthcare facilities should:

- Disclose to consumers factors -- such as methods of compensation, ownership of or interest in healthcare facilities, or matters of conscience -- that could influence advice or treatment decisions.

- Assure that provider contracts do not contain any so-called "gag clauses" or other contractual mechanisms that restrict healthcare providers' ability to communicate with and advise patients about medically necessary treatment options.

- Be prohibited from penalizing or seeking retribution against healthcare professionals or other health workers for advocating on behalf of their patients.

Respect and Nondiscrimination

Consumers have the right to considerate, respectful care from all members of the healthcare industry at all times and under all circumstances. An environment of mutual respect is essential to maintain a quality healthcare system. To assure that right, the Commission recommends the following:

- Consumers must not be discriminated against in the delivery of healthcare services consistent with the benefits covered in their policy, or as required by law, based on race, ethnicity, national origin, religion, sex, age, mental or physical disability, sexual orientation, genetic information, or source of payment.

- Consumers eligible for coverage under the terms and conditions of a health plan or program, or as required by law, must not be discriminated against in marketing and enrollment practices based on race, ethnicity, national origin, religion, sex, age, mental or physical disability, sexual orientation, genetic information, or source of payment.

Confidentiality of Health Information

Consumers have the right to communicate with healthcare providers in confidence and to have the confidentiality of their individually identifiable healthcare information protected. Consumers also have the right to review and copy their own medical records and request amendments to their records.

Complaints and Appeals

Consumers have the right to a fair and efficient process for resolving differences with their health plans, healthcare providers, and the institutions that serve them, including a rigorous system of internal review and an independent system of external review. A free copy of the Patient's Bill of Rights is available from the American Hospital Association.[58]

Patient Responsibilities

Treatment is a two-way street between you and your healthcare providers. To underscore the importance of finance in modern healthcare as well as your responsibility for the financial aspects of your care, the President's Advisory Commission on Consumer Protection and Quality in the Healthcare Industry has proposed that patients understand the following "Consumer Responsibilities."[59] In a healthcare system that protects consumers' rights, it is reasonable to expect and encourage consumers to assume certain responsibilities. Greater individual involvement by the consumer in his or her care increases the likelihood of achieving the best outcome and helps support a quality-oriented, cost-conscious environment. Such responsibilities include:

- Take responsibility for maximizing healthy habits such as exercising, not smoking, and eating a healthy diet.

- Work collaboratively with healthcare providers in developing and carrying out agreed-upon treatment plans.

- Disclose relevant information and clearly communicate wants and needs.

---

[58] To order your free copy of the Patient's Bill of Rights, telephone 312-422-3000 or visit the American Hospital Association's Web site: http://www.aha.org. Click on "Resource Center," go to "Search" at bottom of page, and then type in "Patient's Bill of Rights." The Patient's Bill of Rights is also available from Fax on Demand, at 312-422-2020, document number 471124.

[59] Adapted from http://www.hcqualitycommission.gov/press/cbor.html#head1.

- Use your health insurance plan's internal complaint and appeal processes to address your concerns.

- Avoid knowingly spreading disease.

- Recognize the reality of risks, the limits of the medical science, and the human fallibility of the healthcare professional.

- Be aware of a healthcare provider's obligation to be reasonably efficient and equitable in providing care to other patients and the community.

- Become knowledgeable about your health plan's coverage and options (when available) including all covered benefits, limitations, and exclusions, rules regarding use of network providers, coverage and referral rules, appropriate processes to secure additional information, and the process to appeal coverage decisions.

- Show respect for other patients and health workers.

- Make a good-faith effort to meet financial obligations.

- Abide by administrative and operational procedures of health plans, healthcare providers, and Government health benefit programs.

Choosing an Insurance Plan

There are a number of official government agencies that help consumers understand their healthcare insurance choices.[60] The U.S. Department of Labor, in particular, recommends ten ways to make your health benefits choices work best for you.[61]

1. Your options are important. There are many different types of health benefit plans. Find out which one your employer offers, then check out the plan, or plans, offered. Your employer's human resource office, the health plan administrator, or your union can provide information to help you match your needs and preferences with the available plans. The more information you have, the better your healthcare decisions will be.

2. Reviewing the benefits available. Do the plans offered cover preventive care, well-baby care, vision or dental care? Are there deductibles? Answers to these questions can help determine the out-of-pocket expenses you may

---

[60] More information about quality across programs is provided at the following AHRQ Web site:
http://www.ahrq.gov/consumer/qntascii/qnthplan.htm .
[61] Adapted from the Department of Labor:
http://www.dol.gov/dol/pwba/public/pubs/health/top10-text.html.

face. Matching your needs and those of your family members will result in the best possible benefits. Cheapest may not always be best. Your goal is high quality health benefits.

3. Look for quality. The quality of healthcare services varies, but quality can be measured. You should consider the quality of healthcare in deciding among the healthcare plans or options available to you. Not all health plans, doctors, hospitals and other providers give the highest quality care. Fortunately, there is quality information you can use right now to help you compare your healthcare choices. Find out how you can measure quality. Consult the U.S. Department of Health and Human Services publication "Your Guide to Choosing Quality Health Care" on the Internet at **www.ahcpr.gov/consumer**.

4. Your plan's summary plan description (SPD) provides a wealth of information. Your health plan administrator can provide you with a copy of your plan's SPD. It outlines your benefits and your legal rights under the Employee Retirement Income Security Act (ERISA), the federal law that protects your health benefits. It should contain information about the coverage of dependents, what services will require a co-pay, and the circumstances under which your employer can change or terminate a health benefits plan. Save the SPD and all other health plan brochures and documents, along with memos or correspondence from your employer relating to health benefits.

5. Assess your benefit coverage as your family status changes. Marriage, divorce, childbirth or adoption, and the death of a spouse are all life events that may signal a need to change your health benefits. You, your spouse and dependent children may be eligible for a special enrollment period under provisions of the Health Insurance Portability and Accountability Act (HIPAA). Even without life-changing events, the information provided by your employer should tell you how you can change benefits or switch plans, if more than one plan is offered. If your spouse's employer also offers a health benefits package, consider coordinating both plans for maximum coverage.

6. Changing jobs and other life events can affect your health benefits. Under the Consolidated Omnibus Budget Reconciliation Act (COBRA), you, your covered spouse, and your dependent children may be eligible to purchase extended health coverage under your employer's plan if you lose your job, change employers, get divorced, or upon occurrence of certain other events. Coverage can range from 18 to 36 months depending on your situation. COBRA applies to most employers with 20 or more workers and requires your plan to notify you of your rights. Most plans require eligible individuals to make their COBRA election within 60 days of the plan's notice. Be sure to follow up with your plan sponsor if you don't receive notice, and make sure you respond within the allotted time.

7. HIPAA can also help if you are changing jobs, particularly if you have a medical condition. HIPAA generally limits pre-existing condition exclusions to a maximum of 12 months (18 months for late enrollees). HIPAA also requires this maximum period to be reduced by the length of time you had prior "creditable coverage." You should receive a certificate documenting your prior creditable coverage from your old plan when coverage ends.

8. Plan for retirement. Before you retire, find out what health benefits, if any, extend to you and your spouse during your retirement years. Consult with your employer's human resources office, your union, the plan administrator, and check your SPD. Make sure there is no conflicting information among these sources about the benefits you will receive or the circumstances under which they can change or be eliminated. With this information in hand, you can make other important choices, like finding out if you are eligible for Medicare and Medigap insurance coverage.

9. Know how to file an appeal if your health benefits claim is denied. Understand how your plan handles grievances and where to make appeals of the plan's decisions. Keep records and copies of correspondence. Check your health benefits package and your SPD to determine who is responsible for handling problems with benefit claims. Contact PWBA for customer service assistance if you are unable to obtain a response to your complaint.

10. You can take steps to improve the quality of the healthcare and the health benefits you receive. Look for and use things like Quality Reports and Accreditation Reports whenever you can. Quality reports may contain consumer ratings -- how satisfied consumers are with the doctors in their plan, for instance-- and clinical performance measures -- how well a healthcare organization prevents and treats illness. Accreditation reports provide information on how accredited organizations meet national standards, and often include clinical performance measures. Look for these quality measures whenever possible. Consult "Your Guide to Choosing Quality Health Care" on the Internet at **www.ahcpr.gov/consumer**.

Medicare and Medicaid

Illness strikes both rich and poor families. For low-income families, Medicaid is available to defer the costs of treatment. The Health Care Financing Administration (HCFA) administers Medicare, the nation's largest health insurance program, which covers 39 million Americans. In the following pages, you will learn the basics about Medicare insurance as well as useful contact information on how to find more in-depth information about Medicaid.[62]

Who is Eligible for Medicare?

Generally, you are eligible for Medicare if you or your spouse worked for at least 10 years in Medicare-covered employment and you are 65 years old and a citizen or permanent resident of the United States. You might also qualify for coverage if you are under age 65 but have a disability or End-Stage Renal disease (permanent kidney failure requiring dialysis or transplant). Here are some simple guidelines:

You can get Part A at age 65 without having to pay premiums if:

- You are already receiving retirement benefits from Social Security or the Railroad Retirement Board.

- You are eligible to receive Social Security or Railroad benefits but have not yet filed for them.

- You or your spouse had Medicare-covered government employment.

If you are under 65, you can get Part A without having to pay premiums if:

- You have received Social Security or Railroad Retirement Board disability benefit for 24 months.

- You are a kidney dialysis or kidney transplant patient.

Medicare has two parts:

- Part A (Hospital Insurance). Most people do not have to pay for Part A.

- Part B (Medical Insurance). Most people pay monthly for Part B.

---

[62] This section has been adapted from the Official U.S. Site for Medicare Information: **http://www.medicare.gov/Basics/Overview.asp**.

Part A (Hospital Insurance)

Helps Pay For: Inpatient hospital care, care in critical access hospitals (small facilities that give limited outpatient and inpatient services to people in rural areas) and skilled nursing facilities, hospice care, and some home healthcare.

Cost: Most people get Part A automatically when they turn age 65. You do not have to pay a monthly payment called a premium for Part A because you or a spouse paid Medicare taxes while you were working.

If you (or your spouse) did not pay Medicare taxes while you were working and you are age 65 or older, you still may be able to buy Part A. If you are not sure you have Part A, look on your red, white, and blue Medicare card. It will show "Hospital Part A" on the lower left corner of the card. You can also call the Social Security Administration toll free at 1-800-772-1213 or call your local Social Security office for more information about buying Part A. If you get benefits from the Railroad Retirement Board, call your local RRB office or 1-800-808-0772. For more information, call your Fiscal Intermediary about Part A bills and services. The phone number for the Fiscal Intermediary office in your area can be obtained from the following Web site: **http://www.medicare.gov/Contacts/home.asp**.

Part B (Medical Insurance)

Helps Pay For: Doctors, services, outpatient hospital care, and some other medical services that Part A does not cover, such as the services of physical and occupational therapists, and some home healthcare. Part B helps pay for covered services and supplies when they are medically necessary.

Cost: As of 2001, you pay the Medicare Part B premium of $50.00 per month. In some cases this amount may be higher if you did not choose Part B when you first became eligible at age 65. The cost of Part B may go up 10% for each 12-month period that you were eligible for Part B but declined coverage, except in special cases. You will have to pay the extra 10% cost for the rest of your life.

Enrolling in Part B is your choice. You can sign up for Part B anytime during a 7-month period that begins 3 months before you turn 65. Visit your local Social Security office, or call the Social Security Administration at 1-800-772-1213 to sign up. If you choose to enroll in Part B, the premium is usually taken out of your monthly Social Security, Railroad Retirement, or Civil Service Retirement payment. If you do not receive any of the above payments, Medicare sends you a bill for your part B premium every 3 months. You should receive your Medicare premium bill in the mail by the 10th of the month. If you do not, call the Social Security Administration at 1-800-772-1213, or your local Social Security office. If you get benefits from the Railroad Retirement Board, call your local RRB office or 1-800-808-0772. For more information, call your Medicare carrier about bills and services. The phone number for the Medicare carrier in your area can be found at the following Web site: **http://www.medicare.gov/Contacts/home.asp**. You may have choices in how you get your healthcare including the Original Medicare Plan, Medicare Managed Care Plans (like HMOs), and Medicare Private Fee-for-Service Plans.

Medicaid

Medicaid is a joint federal and state program that helps pay medical costs for some people with low incomes and limited resources. Medicaid programs vary from state to state. People on Medicaid may also get coverage for nursing home care and outpatient prescription drugs which are not covered by Medicare. You can find more information about Medicaid on the HCFA.gov Web site at **http://www.hcfa.gov/medicaid/medicaid.htm**.

States also have programs that pay some or all of Medicare's premiums and may also pay Medicare deductibles and coinsurance for certain people who have Medicare and a low income. To qualify, you must have:

- Part A (Hospital Insurance),

- Assets, such as bank accounts, stocks, and bonds that are not more than $4,000 for a single person, or $6,000 for a couple, and

- A monthly income that is below certain limits.

For more information on these programs, look at the Medicare Savings Programs brochure, **http://www.medicare.gov/Library/PDFNavigation/PDFInterim.asp?Language=English&Type=Pub&PubID=10126**. There are also Prescription Drug Assistance Programs available. Find information on these programs which offer discounts or free medications to individuals in need at **http://www.medicare.gov/Prescription/Home.asp**.

NORD's Medication Assistance Programs

Finally, the National Organization for Rare Disorders, Inc. (NORD) administers medication programs sponsored by humanitarian-minded pharmaceutical and biotechnology companies to help uninsured or under-insured individuals secure life-saving or life-sustaining drugs.[63] NORD programs ensure that certain vital drugs are available "to those individuals whose income is too high to qualify for Medicaid but too low to pay for their prescribed medications." The program has standards for fairness, equity, and unbiased eligibility. It currently covers some 14 programs for nine pharmaceutical companies. NORD also offers early access programs for investigational new drugs (IND) under the approved "Treatment INDs" programs of the Food and Drug Administration (FDA). In these programs, a limited number of individuals can receive investigational drugs that have yet to be approved by the FDA. These programs are generally designed for rare diseases or disorders. For more information, visit **www.rarediseases.org**.

Additional Resources

In addition to the references already listed in this chapter, you may need more information on health insurance, hospitals, or the healthcare system in general. The NIH has set up an excellent guidance Web site that addresses these and other issues. Topics include:[64]

- Health Insurance:
  http://www.nlm.nih.gov/medlineplus/healthinsurance.html

- Health Statistics:
  http://www.nlm.nih.gov/medlineplus/healthstatistics.html

- HMO and Managed Care:
  http://www.nlm.nih.gov/medlineplus/managedcare.html

- Hospice Care: **http://www.nlm.nih.gov/medlineplus/hospicecare.html**

- Medicaid: **http://www.nlm.nih.gov/medlineplus/medicaid.html**

- Medicare: **http://www.nlm.nih.gov/medlineplus/medicare.html**

- Nursing Homes and Long-term Care:
  http://www.nlm.nih.gov/medlineplus/nursinghomes.html

---

[63] Adapted from NORD: **http://www.rarediseases.org/cgi-bin/nord/progserv#patient?id=rPIzL9oD&mv_pc=30**.

[64] You can access this information at:
http://www.nlm.nih.gov/medlineplus/healthsystem.html.

- Patient's Rights, Confidentiality, Informed Consent, Ombudsman Programs, Privacy and Patient Issues:
http://www.nlm.nih.gov/medlineplus/patientissues.html
- Veteran's Health, Persian Gulf War, Gulf War Syndrome, Agent Orange:
http://www.nlm.nih.gov/medlineplus/veteranshealth.html

Vocabulary Builder

Alkaline Phosphatase: An enzyme that catalyzes the conversion of an orthophosphoric monoester and water to an alcohol and orthophosphate. EC 3.1.3.1. [NIH]

Analgesic: An agent that alleviates pain without causing loss of consciousness. [EU]

Arthralgia: Pain in a joint. [EU]

Bronchoscopy: A technique for visualizing the interior of bronchi and instilling or removing fluid or tissue samples by passing a lighted tube (bronchoscope) through the nose or mouth into the bronchi. [NIH]

Hepatomegaly: Enlargement of the liver. [EU]

Hyperpigmentation: Excessive pigmentation of the skin, usually as a result of increased melanization of the epidermis rather than as a result of an increased number of melanocytes. Etiology is varied and the condition may arise from exposure to light, chemicals or other substances, or from a primary metabolic imbalance. [NIH]

Seizures: Clinical or subclinical disturbances of cortical function due to a sudden, abnormal, excessive, and disorganized discharge of brain cells. Clinical manifestations include abnormal motor, sensory and psychic phenomena. Recurrent seizures are usually referred to as epilepsy or "seizure disorder." [NIH]

Splenomegaly: Enlargement of the spleen. [EU]

APPENDIX F. MORE ON THE LUNGS

Overview[65]

Breathing is important because your body needs the oxygen in the air you breathe to create the energy that keeps you alive. Your respiratory system carries the oxygen to your lungs, where it enters your bloodstream to travel throughout your body. This system also carries the "used" air, which is mostly carbon dioxide, back to your lungs so that you can breathe it out.

When fresh air is breathed in through the nose and mouth, it is pulled through the windpipe or trachea and into the lungs. There it moves through two large passageways, called the bronchi. Then a complex system of much smaller tubes or bronchioles branch out to carry oxygen to the "working parts" of the lungs -- millions of air sacs or <u>alveoli</u>. These small sacs (like tiny folded balloons) have very thin walls that are full of blood vessels. The walls are so thin that the oxygen in the air can pass through them to enter your bloodstream and travel to cells in all parts of your body.

In the alveoli, your muscles burn food, using the oxygen you inhale, and create a byproduct gas, carbon dioxide, which is "used" air. Carbon dioxide, is blown out of your body every time you breathe out.

---

[65] From the National Lung Health Education Program: **http://www.nlhep.org/lung.htm#trachea.**

Introduction[66]

Breathing for most of us is something we do without being aware of it. We pay no attention to this continuous activity as we work, play, or sleep. Our lungs are responsible for this essential natural function that gets oxygen into the bloodstream so that it can be delivered to the cells of our body. During a normal day, we breathe nearly 25,000 times. The more than 10,000 liters of air we inhale is mostly oxygen and nitrogen.

In addition, there are small amounts of other gases, floating bacteria, and viruses. It also contains the products of tobacco smoke, automobile exhaust, and other pollutants from the atmosphere in varying amounts. Air pollutants can affect our lungs in many ways. They may simply cause irritation and discomfort. But sometimes inhaled materials can cause illness or death.

The lungs have a series of built-in mechanical and biological barriers that keep harmful materials from entering the body. In addition, specific defense mechanisms can inactivate some disease-causing materials. However, sometimes the normal lung defenses and barriers in the lungs do not work as well as they should. Medical problems at birth or during infancy and growth can affect lung development. Later in life the lungs may be damaged by smoking, occupational exposures, or accidents. These abnormalities allow air pollutants to break through the lung's defenses. The result can be respiratory problems or diseases. This brochure describes the unique structure and functions of the human lung that help maintain respiratory health. It explains how the lungs' inability to carry out their tasks can cause disease or disability. It also lists some simple suggestions for warding off conditions that cause the lungs to malfunction.

The following is offered by the National Heart, Lung, and Blood Institute (NHLBI) together with the National Lung Health Education Program (NLHEP) to meet the common goal of promoting lung health and preventing or reducing lung disease.

The Lungs: A Historical View

Nearly 2,000 years ago, Claudius Galen, a Greek physician, wrote that the lung was an instrument of voice and respiration. He thought that the purpose of respiration was to cool the heart by "the substance of the air." His

---

[66] From NHLBI: **http://www.nhlbi.nih.gov/health/public/lung/other/lungs_hd.pdf**.

concept was that breathing in (inspiration) supplied a cooling substance to the heart while breathing out (expiration) removed hot material from it. At the end of the 16th century, a Dutch scientist, Fabricius, expressed the view that the function of the lungs was to prepare air for the heart. Until the middle of the 17th century, the lungs were thought to be a solid, compact, fleshy mass. At that time Marcello Malpighi, an Italian anatomist, and Thomas Willis, an English clinician, noted independently that the lungs were a system of canals made up of membranes, air passages, and blood vessels. Many of the currently used terms for the components of the lung such as lobules, alveoli, arteries, and veins come from these authors. In 1628, William Harvey, a British physician and physiologist, described his theory of circulation and proposed that the blood was pumped through the lungs by the expansion and contraction of the lungs during breathing. The lungs were once thought to be a solid mass.

Our knowledge about the lungs has come a long way during the more than 300 years since Malpighi, Willis, and Harvey. Today we know that the lungs are a pair of cone-shaped, soft, spongy, pinkish, organs. They get oxygen into the blood and remove carbon dioxide, a waste-product of the body. We have also learned that a major function of the lungs is to protect the body from potentially harmful airborne agents and toxic chemicals that our body may produce. We now know that the lungs have both "respiratory" and "nonrespiratory" functions. The respiratory function of the lungs is "gas exchange." This is the term for the transfer of oxygen from the air into the blood and the removal of carbon dioxide from the blood. The nonrespiratory functions of the lungs are mechanical, bio-chemical, and physiological. The lungs provide the first line of defense against airborne irritants and bacterial, viral, and other infectious agents. They also remove volatile substances and particles of matter generated within the body. The lungs control the flow of water, ions, and large proteins across its various cellular structures. Together with the liver, they remove various products of the body's metabolic reactions. The lungs also manufacture a variety of essential hormones and other chemicals that have precise biological roles.

Human Respiratory System[67]

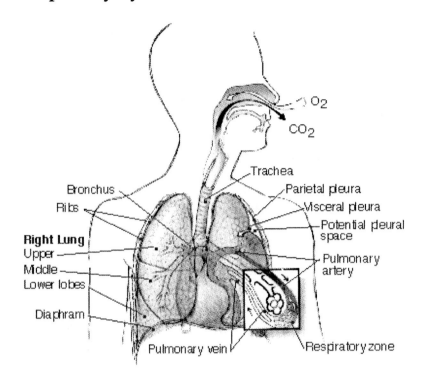

How Do Normal Lungs Work?[68]

Air usually enters the nose and mouth and goes down the air tube (trachea) to two main air passages (bronchi). These passages allow air to go into the right and left lung.

Each bronchus branches out into grape-like air sacs called alveoli. Through the alveoli, oxygen enters the bloodstream during breathing in (inspiration), and carbon dioxide, a waste product, leaves the body during breathing out (expiration).

White blood cells normally found in our bodies help protect us from infection. But white blood cells also release an enzyme, called neutrophil elastase, that can damage the lungs. In normal lungs, alpha-1 antitrypsin protects the lungs from the harmful effects of neutrophil elastase.

---

[67] From NHLBI: **http://www.nhlbi.nih.gov/health/public/lung/other/copd/resp_sys.htm**.
[68] From the NHLBI: **http://www.nhlbi.nih.gov/health/public/lung/other/antitryp.htm**.

Lung Structure and Function: The Big Picture

The lungs are shaped like cones and textured like a fine grained sponge that can be inflated with air. They sit within the thoracic cage where they stretch from the trachea (windpipe) to below the heart. About 10 percent of the lung is solid tissue, the remainder is filled with air and blood. This unique structure of the lung is delicate enough for gas exchange and yet strong enough to maintain its shape and enable it to perform the many functions vital for keeping us healthy.

Two "plumbing" systems, the airways for ventilation (exchange of air between the lungs and the atmosphere) and the circulatory system for perfusion (blood flow), are coordinated by special muscles and nerves. This arrangement enables the lung to perform its primary function of rapidly exchanging oxygen from inhaled air with the carbon dioxide from the blood.

Air enters the body through the nose or the mouth, and travels down the throat and trachea into the chest through a pair of air tubes called bronchi (plural for bronchus). The bronchi divide and subdivide into successive generations of narrower and shorter branching tubes of unequal length and diameter. The final destination for inhaled air is the network of about 3 million air sacs, called alveoli, located at the ends of the lungs' air passages. Between the trachea and alveoli, the lungs look like an inverted tree. The first (main) branching of the trachea leads to the left and right lungs. The two lungs fill most of the chest cavity. Between the lungs are located the heart, the major blood vessels, the trachea, the esophagus (tube leading from the throat to the stomach), and lymph nodes. The thorax (chest wall) surrounds and supports the lungs.

Movement of the air into the lungs is controlled by the respiratory muscles of the thorax. These muscles, collectively called the ventilatory apparatus, include the diaphragm (the muscle that separates the chest and abdominal contents) and the muscles that move the ribs. When the respiratory muscles contract, the chest enlarges like a bellows sucking in air (inhalation). As air fills the lungs they expand automatically. The lungs return to their original (resting) size when we exhale. The performance of the ventilatory apparatus is coordinated by specific nerve sites, called respiratory centers, located in the brain and the neck.

The respiratory centers respond to changes in oxygen, carbon dioxide, and acid levels in the blood. Normal concentrations of these chemicals in arterial blood are maintained by changing the breathing rate. The right lung is slightly larger than the left lung and is divided into three sections or lobes;

the left lung has only two bbes. Each lobe is subdivided into two to five bronchopulmonary segments. The segments are further subdivided into lobules served by smaller branches of the bronchi.

The outside of the lung and the inside of the chest cavity are lined by a single continuous membrane called the pleura. The portion of the pleura surrounding the lungs is called the visceral pleura, while the portion lining the chest cavity is called the parietal pleura. The potential space between the lungs and the inside of the chest cavity is called the pleural space or pleural cavity. The pleural space is moistened with a fluid that lubricates the pleurae as they slide back and forth on each other during ventilation.

Normally the pleural space contains only a small amount of fluid and is free of any gas, blood, or other matter. Blood vessels, bronchi, and nerves come together at the entrance of the lung called the hilum. Bronchopulmonary lymph nodes, important for the drainage of the lungs, are located here. The extensive nervous system of the lungs extends from the hilum to almost all of the lungs' structural units.

The Conducting Airways

The first 16 subdivisions of the bronchi ending in terminal bronchioles are called the conducting airways. Terminal bronchioles are the smallest airways without alveoli. They further divide into respiratory bronchioles, ending in alveolar ducts. Respiratory bronchioles have occassional alveoli budding from their walls, while alveolar ducts are completely lined with alveoli. The last seven branchings of the bronchioles where gas exchange occurs are called the respiratory zone. The terminal respiratory unit of the lung from the respiratory bronchiole to the alveolus is called the acinus.

Gas Exchange

Gas exchange between inhaled air and blood takes place in the alveoli. Blood is brought to the alveoli through a fine network of pulmonary capillaries where it is spread in a thin film. The barrier separating the air and blood is extremely thin, 50 times thinner than a sheet of tissue paper. A large surface area (80 square meters, as large as a tennis court) is available for gas exchange. In the resting state, it takes just about a minute for the total blood volume of the body (about 5 liters) to pass through the lungs. It takes a red cell a fraction of a second to pass through the capillary network. Gas exchange occurs almost instantaneously during this short period.

Cellular and Molecular Aspects

At the cellular and molecular level, the components of the lung are maintained by a unique arrangement of diverse structural proteins and cellular elements. This includes some 40 different types of cells, glands, muscles, and molecules, strategically arranged in intricate but orderly patterns in various parts of the lung.

The controlled complexity of the various parts of the lungs facilitates their many functions. Oxygen-poor blood is pumped from the right ventricle of the heart through a system of pulmonary arteries, arterioles, and capillaries to the alveoli, and the oxygen-rich blood is returned to the left heart through a collecting system of venules and veins. This extensive system, called the pulmonary circulation, filters clots, fat particles, and cellular debris from the bloodstream. It also moves liquid and large and small molecules across the pulmonary blood vessels, providing oxygen and nutrients, and facilitating various metabolic functions of the lung including the synthesis of substances such as surfactant. The lungs also have a second blood supply from the bronchial circulation.

The purpose of this blood supply is to provide nutrients especially for the large airways. Bronchial circulation represents only a small portion (1-2 percent) of the cardiac output. In this system, bronchial arteries bring oxygenated blood from the left side of the heart to the airways (bronchi, bronchioles) and the supporting structures (connective tissue) of the lung. Bronchial venous blood is returned, just like the venous blood from the rest of the body, to the right atrium.

Bronchial circulation is believed to be more important in the fetal lung than in the adult lung. Conducting airways receive their blood supply from branches of bronchial arteries, while the terminal respiratory units receive blood from branches of the pulmonary arteries. Gas exchange occurs by diffusion of gases across the alveolar membranes into and out of the blood as it flows through the capillaries. Oxygen-poor blood discards its carbon dioxide into the alveoli, and hemoglobin, an oxygen-carrying protein in the red blood cells, binds with oxygen from inhaled air (becomes "arterialized").

Although the red blood cells are exposed to alveolar air only for a fraction of a second, gas exchange between alveoli and capillaries takes place very efficiently because there is an extremely large surface area between the blood and the air. The bronchi contain specialized connective tissue (cartilage), while bronchioles are noncartilaginous.

The bronchi mostly serve nonrespiratory roles such as ridding the airways of irritating particles; their only respiratory function is to carry air from the external environment to the distal sites of gas exchange. The arteries and capillaries that bring blood to the alveoli are lined with a layer of delicate specialized cells called endothelial cells. The air-blood barrier is composed of three tissue layers — an endothelium lining the capillaries; an epithelium lining the airspaces; and, between them, an interstitial layer composed of connective tissue, interstitial extracellular matrix, and mesenchymal cells. The interstitial layer also contains special cells — alveolar macrophages, lymphocytes, and inflammatory cells — that can defend or injure the lungs, depending on the situation. Dispersed throughout the interstitium are proteins, lipids, carbohydrates, and other substances derived from plasma and cells. The endothelium acts as a barrier retarding the passage of fluid, proteins, and other blood components from the vessel lumen into the interstitium and air spaces of the lung. In addition, the endothelial cells perform many of the nonrespiratory functions of the lung, particularly the transformation of a variety of bioactive substances. The walls of the conducting airways are mostly composed of epithelial lining, connective tissue elements, and a smooth muscle sleeve.

The exact proportion of these constituents varies depending on whether the walls are in the large bronchi, the bronchioles, or the alveoli. The epithelium also contains unique mixtures of cells with distinct functions. These functions vary depending on the level of the airway at which the cells are located.

The lungs' first line of defense against injury from inhaled agents is a mix of anatomic barriers, nonspecific mechanical and cellular defenses, antimicrobial secretions, and circulating and resident scavenger (phagocytic) cells that engulf or digest particulates. Removal of particles from the conducting airways (nose to respiratory bronchioles) is carried out by "mucociliary clearance," helped by airway secretions. A film of mucus produced in the lungs envelops the particles which are then continuously moved by the rhythmic beating motions of cilia (hair-like structures that extend from the surface of the cells) to the oropharynx where they are swallowed or coughed out. These defenses are present at birth.

Operating beyond the nonspecific defenses, are specific acquired immune mechanisms that are latent until activated by natural (maternal transfer or infections) or artificial exposures (vaccinations) to foreign materials. These highly specific defenses of the lung are initiated by complex interactions between foreign substances (antigens) and specialized cells.

These interactions result in antibody-mediated or cell-mediated immunities that provide uniquely specific defenses against certain organisms or agents. Research supported by the National Heart, Lung, and Blood Institute is generating new knowledge on previously unrecognized physiological and metabolic processes and mediators operating in the lung. Scientists now realize that the lung, an organ once thought to be merely an inert balloon serving as a receptacle for air, is in reality a powerhouse of concerted and interrelated mechanical, physiological, neurological, immunological, pharmacological, and metabolic functions necessary to sustain life.

APPENDIX G. MORE ON LUNG DISEASES

Overview[69]

Estimates of the number of known lung diseases vary from a few dozen to several hundred. Lung diseases are classified and counted either as individual, specific diseases, or as groups of diseases that share common features. These features may be their sites, etiologies (initiating events), pathophysiology (abnormalities of function), or clinical features (signs and symptoms). Most doctors find it convenient to deal with lung diseases in groups, based on the particular pulmonary (lung) component that is diseased. Examples are diseases of the airways, diseases of the interstitium (the space between tissues), or disorders of the pulmonary circulation, the ventilatory apparatus, or gas exchange. Often, many of these diseases occur together, particularly if they are caused by infection, inflammation, or cancer. In such cases they present an overlapping, progressive series of a mixture of clinical symptoms.

How Do Normal Lungs Work?[70]

Air usually enters the nose and mouth and goes down the air tube (trachea) to two main air passages (bronchi). These passages allow air to go into the right and left lung.

Each bronchus branches out into grape-like air sacs called alveoli. Through the alveoli, oxygen enters the bloodstream during breathing in (inspiration),

---

[69] From the National Lung Health Education Program:
http://www.nlhep.org/lung.htm#trachea.
[70] From the NHLBI: **http://www.nhlbi.nih.gov/health/public/lung/other/antitryp.htm** .

and carbon dioxide, a waste product, leaves the body during breathing out (expiration).

White blood cells normally found in our bodies help protect us from infection. But white blood cells also release an enzyme, called neutrophil elastase, that can damage the lungs. In normal lungs, alpha-1 antitrypsin protects the lungs from the harmful effects of neutrophil elastase.

Lung Diseases: How They Begin

The most common clinical signs of lung diseases are cough, chest pain, chest tightness, shortness of breath (dyspnea), and abnormal breathing patterns. When any of these symptoms appear, it may signal that some vital functions of the lung have been disturbed. Because most individuals have enormous reserves of lung tissue, the disturbances in lung defenses or function may have begun some time before the clinical symptoms begin to appear. Some lung disorders are caused by general diseases of muscles or nervous systems.

Respiratory problems can have a number of causes. They usually arise from acute or chronic inhalation of toxic agents in the workplace or other settings, accidents, or harmful lifestyles such as smoking. Infections, genetic factors, or anything else that directly or indirectly affects lung development and function can also cause respiratory symptoms. In some lung diseases, the lung itself has been damaged. Others result from diseases of the nervous system or the muscles. These disorders interfere with the normal function of the respiratory muscles so that, although the lung itself is normal, breathing is difficult.

Diseases of the Airways

Airways diseases are lung disorders that are primarily due to a continuing obstruction of airflow. Acute or chronic airflow obstruction or limitation can be caused by a variety of structural changes in the airways. Asthma, chronic bronchitis, emphysema, bronchiolitis, cystic fibrosis, and bronchiectasis are some common airways diseases. The term chronic obstructive pulmonary disease (COPD) is commonly used for chronic bronchitis and emphysema that exist together in many patients and in which the airway obstruction is mostly irreversible. COPD is the fourth most common and the most rapidly increasing cause of death in the United States. In asthma, reversible airway obstruction is caused by inflammation, contraction of the airway smooth muscle, increased mucus secretion, and plugging of the bronchioles.

In chronic bronchitis, airway obstruction results from chronic and excessive secretion of abnormal airway mucus, inflammation, bronchospasm, and infections.

In emphysema, a structural element (elastin) in the terminal bronchioles is destroyed leading to collapse of the airway walls and inability to exhale "stale" air.

Bronchiolitis in children is due to viral infections that cause obstructive inflammatory changes in the bronchioles.

In bronchiolitis obliterans (obliteration of bronchioles, occurring in transplanted lung or after bone marrow transplantation), inflammatory changes that occur in transplanted lungs eventually cause blocking of the lumen (air channel) of the bronchioles; this is a sign that the new lung is being rejected.

Cystic fibrosis is a genetic disease in which thickened airway mucus, pulmonary infections, and inflammation lead to bronchiectasis and airway obstruction.

In bronchiectasis, airway obstruction is due to chronic abnormal dilation (stretching) of the bronchi and the destruction of the elastic and muscular components of the bronchial walls; it is usually caused by repeated lung infections.

Diseases of the Interstitium

The interstitium (the space between tissues) of the lungs includes portions of the connective tissue of the blood vessels and air sacs. Major chronic diseases of the lower respiratory tract in which fibrosis (scarring of the lung tissue) occurs affect the interstitial tissue. Sarcoidosis and pulmonary fibrosis are examples of the more than 150 interstitial lung diseases. Another term for these diseases is "stiff lung" disease. The most common symptoms are shortness of breath after exercise and a nonproductive cough. Some patients with interstitial lung diseases have fever, fatigue, muscle and joint pain, and abnormal chest sounds. As these diseases advance, heart function is affected. Some interstitial lung diseases are caused by occupational or environmental exposure to inorganic dusts. Workers who inhale particles of silica are at risk for silicosis; similarly, workers in beryllium mines may develop berylliosis.

Interstitial lung diseases may also be caused by inhaling organic dusts such as bacteria. Lung disease that results from breathing in animal proteins is called hypersensitivity pneumonitis. Drugs, poisons, infections, and radiation have also been known to cause these diseases. However, approximately two-thirds of the cases of interstitial lung diseases have no known cause and are therefore termed "idiopathic." Interstitial lung diseases begin with inflammation of the lung cells. This may be caused by an immune response or injury. The lungs stiffen as a result of inflammation of the air sacs (alveolitis) and scarring (fibrosis).

Disorders of Gas Exchange and Blood Circulation

Pulmonary edema occurs when excess fluid collects in the tissues and air spaces of the lungs. The fluid interferes with gas exchange, thus causing the patient to be short of breath and to possibly have wheezing and a persistent cough. Pulmonary edema may result from diseases of the heart or may occur as complications of other illnesses such as widespread viral or other infections, drug toxicity, exposure to high altitudes, kidney failure, or hemorrhagic shock.

Pulmonary embolism is the sudden blocking of the blood flow in one of the arteries in the lung. The highly branched network of blood vessels in the lung filters the blood as it flows through it. Sometimes the blood carries a blood clot, a fat globule, an air bubble, or a piece of tissue that is large enough to block a blood vessel leading to the lung's network of capillaries. Gas exchange then can no longer occur in this section of the lung. The result is shortness of breath or even heart failure.

The most common form of pulmonary embolism is a thromboembolism. It occurs when a blood clot travels from the legs or pelvis to the pulmonary blood vessels. Respiratory failure is the inability of the lungs to perform gas exchange. It occurs either when the muscles of the ventilatory system fail or when the structures that perform gas exchange are unable to function. Patients with neuromuscular diseases such as muscular dystrophy and polio may have normal lungs, but they can develop respiratory failure because their disease-weakened muscles are unable to pump air into their lungs. When gas exchange is impaired, not enough oxygen gets into the blood to fuel the body's metabolic activity. This condition is called hypoxemia. Chronic hypoxemia causes the blood vessels in the lung to contract; the result is pulmonary hypertension. Hypoxemia may also weaken the heart and the circulatory system. Any lung disease, if not adequately treated, can lead to respiratory failure.

Adult or acute respiratory distress syndrome (ARDS) was once called "shock lung." It is a type of pulmonary edema that is not related to heart problems. It has many causes such as severe infections, exposure to toxic fumes, circulatory collapse, sepsis (presence of disease-causing organisms or their toxic products in blood or other tissues), shock following severe blood loss, and bone fractures. During ARDS, there is severe damage to the alveolar surfaces, the blood-air barrier becomes leaky, and protein- containing fluid fills the alveoli so that they can no longer conduct gas exchange.

Respiratory distress syndrome of the newborn (RDS) is a type of respiratory failure that develops most commonly in premature or low birth weight babies whose lungs have not yet made enough surfactant. The surfactant is critical for opening the baby's alveoli with its first breath and keeping them open. As the lungs collapse, respiratory distress occurs. Pulmonary hypertension is a disorder in which the blood pressure in the pulmonary arteries is abnormally high. In severe pulmonary hypertension, the right side of the heart must work harder than usual to pump blood against the high pressure. When this continues for long periods, the right heart enlarges and functions poorly, and fluid collects in the ankles (edema) and the belly. Eventually the left side of the heart begins to fail. Heart failure caused by pulmonary disease is called cor pulmonale. The most common causes of cor pulmonale are various combinations of emphysema, chronic bronchitis, and/or fibrosis. When pulmonary hypertension occurs in the absence of any other disease, it is called primary pulmonary hypertension. It affects more women than men; its cause is not known.

Pulmonary hypertension that results from another disease of the heart or lungs (for example, congenital heart disease, pulmonary thromboembolism, COPD, or interstitial fibrosis) is called secondary pulmonary hypertension. Lung Disorders From Unusual Atmospheric Pressure At high altitudes, the air pressure is less than at sea level, and the air contains less oxygen. Some individuals traveling to high altitudes experience a variety of symptoms while they adapt to changes in the atmosphere. The symptoms are probably due to excess fluid accumulation in the tissues. n Acute mountain sickness causes dizziness, headache, and drowsiness; lethargy, shortness of breath, and nausea and vomiting may also occur.

High altitude cerebral edema (fluid in brain tissue) is diagnosed when a person has symptoms of severe headache, confusion, nausea, and vomiting. Seizures may occur that can lead to coma and even death.

High altitude pulmonary edema (fluid in the lung tissue) may cause cough and shortness of breath on exercise or, when severe, progressive shortness of breath even at rest, suffocation, and death.

When people dive into deep water below sea level, they become exposed to increased atmospheric pressures. This causes greater than normal amounts of nitrogen to become dissolved in their blood. If the diver returns too quickly to the surface, the excess nitrogen leaves the blood in the form of bubbles that lodge in the blood vessels of vital organs, causing necrosis (cell death) in surrounding tissue. Although this condition (decompression sickness) typically involves the limbs near a joint and is known as the bends, it can also occur in the chest, lung, or brain.

Disorders of the Pleura

Pleural effusion means an accumulation of fluid in the pleural space. It may result from heart failure, cancer, pulmonary embolism, or inflammation. If the pleurae themselves are inflamed, the condition is called pleurisy. Pleurisy causes severe chest pain with every breath and may occur with pleural effusion. If blood is the accumulating fluid, the condition is referred to as hemothorax. If the accumulating liquid is pus, it is called empyema. When air accumulates in the pleural spaces, the condition is called pneumothorax. Mechanical injuries or diffuse diseases of the lung that distort lung architecture can lead to pneumothorax. Such diseases include emphysema, asthma, and cystic fibrosis. The most common symptom of pneumothorax is sudden pain on one side of the lung accompanied by shortness of breath.

Infections

Infections are a major cause of respiratory illness. They can be caused by bacteria or viruses and can affect not only the lung but also the nose, sinuses, ears, teeth, and gums. Infections may also complicate other lung diseases. Pneumonia, or inflammation of the lungs, is the most common type of infectious disease of the lung. Infectious pneumonias are usually identified by naming the cause of the infection or the pattern of the infection in the respiratory tract. More than half the cases of pneumonia are caused by the bacterium, Streptococcal pneumoniae (pneumococcus) and are called pneumococcal pneumonia. Influenza A is the cause of a significant number of cases of pneumonia in the elderly during the winter months. Another well-known form of pneumonia is Legionnaires' disease, which is caused by the organism, Legionella pneumophila. The inflammatory response of the lung in pneumonia varies depending on the type of infection, and might include:

- Lobar consolidation: solidification of the lung as air spaces are filled with fluid and cellular material, and

- Interstitial inflammation.

Pneumonia is sometimes accompanied by:

- Necrosis: tissue changes accompanying cell death, - cavitation: hollow spaces walled off by scar tissue,

- Abscess: pus formation, and

- Granuloma formation: production of tumor-like masses of different kinds of cells due to a chronic inflammatory response. Tuberculosis is a granulomatous infectious disease caused by an organism called mycobacterium tuberculosis.

Early Symptoms of Breathing Problems[71]

Early discovery of a breathing problem and appropriate treatment can prevent the disease from progressing to the point that it seriously affects the way you live and work.

Anyone who has an ongoing cough or shortness of breath, even if it seems minor, should see his or her doctor. Morning cough, for example, is not normal. It is a result of smoking and indicates that there is irritation and swelling within the lung. Shortness of breath while exercising, climbing stairs, or walking can also be a sign of a breathing problem. Many people simply feel that they are "out of shape," slowing down, or getting older when, in fact, they are working harder to breathe.

A spirometer can tell whether your breathing is normal. It takes only a couple of minutes to blow into this machine, which can detect a change in your breathing ability even before you do. Fortunately, many physicians

---

[71] From the National Lung Health Education Program: **http://www.nlhep.org/lung.htm#trachea**.

have a spirometer in their offices. The next time you see a doctor, ask for a spirometry test if you think you might have COPD or asthma.

Another very simple test can be done with a peak-flow meter. This device measures the openness of the airways or airflow and can detect small changes before symptoms appear. A peak-flow meter can be used to monitor airflow at home or at work.

Who Should Have a Breathing Test?

- Does asthmatic bronchitis, chronic bronchitis or emphysema run in your family?

- Do you smoke?

- Are you short of breath more often than other people?

- Do you cough?

- When you cough, do you cough up yellow or green mucus?

If the answer to any of the above questions is yes, you should see your doctor for a breathing test. After taking the test, you can ask your doctor these questions:

- Are my breathing measurements normal or abnormal?

- How abnormal are they?

- Is the problem one that can be treated with drugs and/or by stopping smoking?

- Is the abnormality worsening? If so, how quickly?

- What exactly should I do for my problem?

Diagnosing Lung Diseases[72]

When a person's symptoms suggest lung disease, a chest x ray is usually the first examination the doctor orders. Then various tests are performed to identify the disease and to determine how severe it is. These tests include:

- Pulmonary function tests;

- Microscopic examination of lung tissue, cells, and fluids using a light microscope and an electron microscope; and

---

[72] From NHLBI: **http://www.nhlbi.nih.gov/health/public/lung/other/lungs_hd.pdf**.

- Biochemical and cellular studies of respiratory fluids removed from the lung by lavage (washing).

To determine how well the lungs are working, doctors can measure respiratory or gas exchange functions, airway or bronchial activity, particle clearance rates, and permeability of the blood-air barrier.

Spirometry

Spirometry, like the measurement of blood pressure, is useful for assessing lung function as well as general health. It is the simplest and most common of the lung function tests. Spirometry measures how much and how quickly air can be expelled following a deep breath. It is performed by having the patient breathe out forcefully into a device called a spirometer. At the same time a machine makes a tracing of the rate at which the air leaves the lung.

Diseases of airflow obstruction and of lung stiffening give characteristic tracings with spirometry. Measures of the amount of air that can be expelled following a deep breath, forced vital capacity (FVC), and the amount of air that can be forcibly exhaled in 1 second, forced expiratory volume in 1 second (FEV 1), are the most useful numbers derived from spirometry. The ratio of FEV 1 to FVC is often used to assess patients for airflow obstruction. It is normally 75 to 85 percent, depending on the patient's age. The ratio is reduced in obstructive diseases, while it is preserved or even increased in restrictive disorders.

A lower than normal FEV 1 is a sign that a lung disease is present. A falling FEV 1 is a sign that a person's lung disease is getting worse. The "normal" values for FVC and FEV 1 for a patient depend on the individual's age, gender, height, and race. They are higher for younger than for older people, higher for tall than for short individuals, higher for men than for women, and higher for whites than blacks or Asians. Therefore, the numbers are presented as percentages of the average expected in someone of the same age, height, sex, and race. This is called percent predicted.

Any number smaller than 85 percent of predicted is considered abnormal. If these numbers are abnormal, the patient is referred for additional pulmonary function tests to find out why. These may include checking the patient's response to bronchodilators, absolute lung volumes, and blood levels of oxygen and carbon dioxide which tell how well gas exchange is occurring. Other important measures of lung function are arterial blood gas tensions (PaO 2 and PaCO 2) and the diffusing capacity of the lung for carbon monoxide (DLCO). Some doctors recommend having spirometry before age 25 to get baseline numbers. However, if you are a smoker, are occupationally exposed to irritants, or have symptoms of cough, wheeze, or shortness of breath, you should be checked with a spirometer at intervals of 3 to 5 years or more frequently if your doctor recommends it. Smokers should have spirometry done at least every 3 to 5 years.

Abnormal spirometry numbers at any age means that you are at risk for early lung disease and even potentially fatal lung cancer, heart disease, or stroke. You should immediately stop smoking if you still smoke, and talk to your doctor about other measures you may need to take depending on the reasons for your abnormal numbers. PREVENTING LUNG DISEASES

Treatment[73]

What can you do if you have an early stage of asthmatic bronchitis, chronic bronchitis, or emphysema? Certainly you should change any behavior that can make it worse. The single most important thing you can do for yourself is to stop smoking. In fact, if you don't stop smoking, none of your other efforts will be as effective as they could be, and your COPD will get worse.

As a COPD patient, you need clean air. Therefore, you should also avoid being around smokers and fume-laden air. During fog or smog, try to stay indoors with windows closed. If possible, fumeless appliances should be used for heating.

Polluted air also can irritate your breathing passages. Try not to go out when the air quality is rated poor. But if you cannot avoid excessive air pollution, protecting your mouth and nose with a mask may improve your breathing.

You should see your doctor on a regular basis and especially if you have a chest cold or any time you cough up mucus. It is also important to guard against catching the flu by getting an influenza vaccine each fall, well before winter starts. A pneumonia vaccine should also be given to anyone over age 60, and all persons with COPD.

There are many different types of treatments that can help you cope with a chronic lung disease and live your life to the fullest. Next, we will discuss

---

[73] From the National Lung Health Education Program: http://www.nlhep.org/lung.htm#trachea.

some of these treatments. Your doctor will select the ones that will be helpful for you.

Clearing Your Lungs

Coughing has an important "cleaning action" and is something you should do every morning and evening. You must learn to cough in such a way that you can clear your lungs of mucus with two or three coughs. There are many ways to do this; your doctor will teach you the way that is best for your particular problem.

As an aid to this cleaning, your doctor might recommend breathing moist or humid air, and drinking plenty of fluids every day. This helps to thin out the mucus so that you can cough it up more easily.

Your doctor might also recommend inhaled bronchodilating drugs or antiinflammatory drugs that open your airways and help increase the normal flow of mucus out of your lungs.

Breathing Techniques

Learning to breathe properly is another very important lesson for people with asthmatic bronchitis, chronic bronchitis, or emphysema. If you have COPD, you usually work very hard to breathe. However, because you are not breathing properly, your hard work does not make you feel better and you become tired easily.

There are several things you can do to improve your breathing:

- First, it is important to relax. You must be relaxed when you breathe.
- Breathe out against pursed lips, like when whistling. This slows down the number of breaths you take. This allows each breath to do more good for you.
- Lean forward while exercising. This also helps stop shortness of breath.
- "Belly breathing" will also help shortness of breath. This is done by allowing your belly to stick out while breathing in and then pulling your belly in while breathing out against pursed lips.

Physical Activity

Often people make the mistake of believing that if they try to avoid becoming short of breath, they will protect their lungs and heart. Nothing could be less true. Remaining physically active will improve your breathing ability and help you feel better and enjoy life more.

You can learn how to exercise more even if you have COPD. As we all know, muscles will become weak if we don't use them. This is true for the muscles of your chest, which are important in breathing, as well. Strengthening these muscles will help stop shortness of breath.

Don't let COPD change your normal attitudes about exercise. You should walk every day, going farther each day than you did the one before. First, walk in your house, then out of doors -- walking longer distances each time. You will soon notice that you are breathing better because using the muscles in your chest helps stop shortness of breath.

Your doctor will tell you which exercises are best for you and plan an exercise program based upon your ability. Ask about local pulmonary programs.

Oxygen

Oxygen is a very helpful treatment that enables many patients with severe COPD to lead a more normal and productive life. If your doctor feels your body is not getting enough oxygen, he or she may prescribe it for you. Portable cylinders will allow you to carry oxygen with you, or your doctor might tell you to use it at night during sleep when a lack of oxygen is most severe. Liquid portable oxygen is the most practical ambulatory system. Your doctor must order the proper oxygen system which can benefit you the most. A supplier cannot change your doctor's prescription. Follow the directions you are given carefully, as you would for any medication that is prescribed.

Mist-Generating Devices

This type of treatment, which must be prescribed by your doctor, delivers a mist of medication and moisture to your lungs. The device that is most often used to create this mist is a "pump-driven nebulizer." The liquid medication is placed in the nebulizer where it is changed into a mist that you inhale. When taking this treatment, here are some points to remember:

- Be sure you know the amount of medication and solution to use as well as the length and timing of your treatment. Follow your doctor's or respiratory therapist's instructions carefully about when each treatment should be scheduled and the length of time that it should be done.

- Relax and sit in a comfortable chair in an upright position.

- Make sure the tubing is not bent or dented, and that the handhold is at the same level as your mouth.

- Put the mouthpiece in front of your teeth and keep your mouth slightly open.

- Take a deep, slow breath and activate the nebulizer control. Let the mist fill your lungs. Hold your breath for about two seconds before exhaling. Remember to exhale slowly and completely each time.

- If your mouth becomes dry during your treatment, don't be afraid to stop and drink some water. Also -- and this is very important -- if you bring up mucus during the treatment, turn your machine off and stop and cough it up. These treatments are helpful in eliminating mucus.

If you experience any discomfort after treatment, notify your doctor.

Medications

Many different medications are used as treatment for asthmatic bronchitis, chronic bronchitis, or emphysema. Your doctor will decide which medicine is best for you based on your medical history, breathing tests, and laboratory tests.

To help you breathe easier, your doctor may give you bronchodilator drugs. Bronchodilators relax the muscles that surround the breathing tubes and widen them, letting air travel in and out more easily.

Your doctor may also prescribe drugs to liquefy the mucus in your lungs, or even drugs called steroids, which reduce the swelling in your breathing tubes. If you have an infection in your respiratory system, your medications may include antibiotics.

These medications may be available in many different forms. In addition to pills or syrups, your doctor may prescribe a metered-dose inhaler, which has medication that you breathe in. Liquid medications may be used with special equipment that will turn them into a mist that will provide moisture for your respiratory system. This mist-maker is called a nebulizer. It is discussed below.

Metered-Dose Inhalers

Most of these devices, which deliver medication to your lungs as a spray, require a prescription from your doctor. The medication in a metered-dose inhaler that can be bought without a prescription such as Primatine Mist™ is adrenaline, a short-acting drug which may be dangerous for persons with heart disease. It is inadequate to treat COPD.

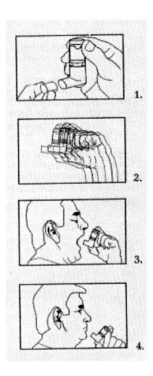

In order to get the maximum benefit from the medication, it is important that the inhaler be used properly. Here are some helpful tips for using a metered-dose inhaler:

- Remove the cap from the mouthpiece.

- Shake the inhaler for a few seconds. Breathe out.

- Hold the inhaler upright and place it in front of your mouth. Keep your mouth slightly open. Breathe in deeply and at the same time press the inhaler between your thumb and forefinger. This will force the medication from the inhaler into your throat and lungs.

- Remove the inhaler and hold your breath for a few seconds; then resume normal breathing. Wait at least two minutes before repeating the process. (Most inhaler medications specify that two puffs should be taken. Wait at least two minutes between each puff.)

Do not exceed the dose prescribed by your doctor. If you continue to have difficulty breathing, contact your doctor immediately.

A device called a spacer or volume chamber should also be used to make it easier to take your medication. This device catches the mist produced by a metered-dose inhaler and holds it so that you can breathe it in at a slower rate.

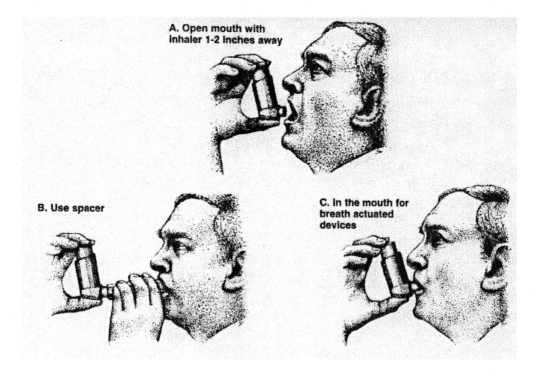

New Developments in Treatment

Progress is continually being made in the treatment of asthmatic bronchitis, chronic bronchitis, and emphysema. Another type of bronchodilator medication (an anticholinergic), is available in metered-dose devices. The other major type of inhaled bronchodilator is called a beta agonist. Beta agonist medications are also available as solutions for use with pump-driven nebulizers. Anticholinergic solutions are also useful in COPD. Both medications can be used together in the same nebulizer. Both are sold in a metered-dose inhaler (separately and mixed together for convenience). Since these bronchodilators work on the respiratory system in different ways, they can be used together to treat COPD.

A new treatment that may be effective in a rare hereditary form of emphysema is being tested on volunteers. A replacement for the inherited deficiency of alpha antitrypsin is commercially available. Although it restores a protective material in the lungs, its effectiveness in preventing the progress of emphysema remains to be proven.

Surgical approaches to improving dyspnea by removing areas of major lung damage from emphysema are called lung volume reduction surgery, (LVRS). In selected patients, this operation can improve shortness of breath and quality of life. The mechanisms behind this improvement are complex. They include a restoration of the curvature of the diaphragm through a reduction in overinflation of diseased parts of the lung. These regions of excessive destruction are often in the upper parts of the lung, (apices). These areas contribute little to lung function, but they take up a lot of space for expansion of the rest of the lung, which is relatively normal. Extensive evaluations must be done through scans and tests of heart function to determine good candidates. At the present time, Medicare does not reimburse for this operation, pending the results of a study. This study contrasts the results from surgery following a period of pulmonary rehabilitation compared to pulmonary rehabilitation alone. This study is known as the National Emphysema Therapy Trial, (NETT). It will be five years or more before the results of NETT are known. Qualified surgeons are presently offering this operation to selected patients on an individual basis when patients have financing resources outside of Medicare. Patients should be evaluated by pulmonologists and surgeons, working together before going ahead with this treatment.

The Future

Today doctors and scientists have a better understanding than ever of the nature of asthmatic bronchitis, chronic bronchitis, and emphysema. These diseases are viewed as damage to the lungs as a result of two factors:

- First, the hereditary loss of certain lung defenses, which leaves lungs more vulnerable to damage.

- The second factor is outside conditions such as smoking, air and environmental pollution, and in some cases, frequent infections.

The future promises more advances in understanding why patients get asthmatic bronchitis, chronic bronchitis, and emphysema.

Diagnosing any breathing problem at an early stage is most important. The treatments and medications discussed in this document can help stop the progress of COPD, in addition to making your life as comfortable as possible. The earlier this is done, the better your health will be.

ONLINE GLOSSARIES

The Internet provides access to a number of free-to-use medical dictionaries and glossaries. The National Library of Medicine has compiled the following list of online dictionaries:

- ADAM Medical Encyclopedia (A.D.A.M., Inc.), comprehensive medical reference: **http://www.nlm.nih.gov/medlineplus/encyclopedia.html**

- MedicineNet.com Medical Dictionary (MedicineNet, Inc.): **http://www.medterms.com/Script/Main/hp.asp**

- Merriam-Webster Medical Dictionary (Inteli-Health, Inc.): **http://www.intelihealth.com/IH/**

- Multilingual Glossary of Technical and Popular Medical Terms in Eight European Languages (European Commission) - Danish, Dutch, English, French, German, Italian, Portuguese, and Spanish: **http://allserv.rug.ac.be/~rvdstich/eugloss/welcome.html**

- On-line Medical Dictionary (CancerWEB): **http://www.graylab.ac.uk/omd/**

- Technology Glossary (National Library of Medicine) - Health Care Technology: **http://www.nlm.nih.gov/nichsr/ta101/ta10108.htm**

- Terms and Definitions (Office of Rare Diseases): **http://rarediseases.info.nih.gov/ord/glossary_a-e.html**

Beyond these, MEDLINEplus contains a very user-friendly encyclopedia covering every aspect of medicine (licensed from A.D.A.M., Inc.). The ADAM Medical Encyclopedia Web site address is **http://www.nlm.nih.gov/medlineplus/encyclopedia.html**. ADAM is also available on commercial Web sites such as Web MD **(http://my.webmd.com/adam/asset/adam_disease_articles/a_to_z/a)** and drkoop.com **(http://www.drkoop.com/)**. Topics of interest can be researched by using keywords before continuing elsewhere, as these basic definitions and concepts will be useful in more advanced areas of research. You may choose to print various pages specifically relating to sarcoidosis and keep them on file. The NIH, in particular, suggests that patients with sarcoidosis visit the following Web sites in the ADAM Medical Encyclopedia:

- **Basic Guidelines for Sarcoidosis**

  Erythema nodosum
  Web site:
  http://www.nlm.nih.gov/medlineplus/ency/article/000881.htm

  Sarcoidosis
  Web site:
  http://www.nlm.nih.gov/medlineplus/ency/article/000076.htm

- **Signs & Symptoms for Sarcoidosis**

  Armpit lump
  Web site:
  http://www.nlm.nih.gov/medlineplus/ency/article/003099.htm

  Arthralgia
  Web site:
  http://www.nlm.nih.gov/medlineplus/ency/article/003261.htm

  Blindness
  Web site:
  http://www.nlm.nih.gov/medlineplus/ency/article/003040.htm

  Breath sounds
  Web site:
  http://www.nlm.nih.gov/medlineplus/ency/article/003323.htm

  Chest discomfort
  Web site:
  http://www.nlm.nih.gov/medlineplus/ency/article/003079.htm

  Cough
  Web site:
  http://www.nlm.nih.gov/medlineplus/ency/article/003072.htm

  Difficulty breathing
  Web site:
  http://www.nlm.nih.gov/medlineplus/ency/article/003075.htm

Dyspnea
Web site:
http://www.nlm.nih.gov/medlineplus/ency/article/003075.htm

Enlarged liver
Web site:
http://www.nlm.nih.gov/medlineplus/ency/article/003275.htm

Enlarged lymph glands
Web site:
http://www.nlm.nih.gov/medlineplus/ency/article/003097.htm

Enlarged spleen
Web site:
http://www.nlm.nih.gov/medlineplus/ency/article/003276.htm

Eye burning, itching and discharge
Web site:
http://www.nlm.nih.gov/medlineplus/ency/article/003034.htm

Fatigue
Web site:
http://www.nlm.nih.gov/medlineplus/ency/article/003088.htm

Fever
Web site:
http://www.nlm.nih.gov/medlineplus/ency/article/003090.htm

General ill feeling
Web site:
http://www.nlm.nih.gov/medlineplus/ency/article/003089.htm

Hair loss
Web site:
http://www.nlm.nih.gov/medlineplus/ency/article/003246.htm

Headache
Web site:
http://www.nlm.nih.gov/medlineplus/ency/article/003024.htm

Hepatomegaly
Web site:
http://www.nlm.nih.gov/medlineplus/ency/article/003275.htm

Hyperpigmentation
Web site:
http://www.nlm.nih.gov/medlineplus/ency/article/003242.htm

Itching
Web site:
http://www.nlm.nih.gov/medlineplus/ency/article/003217.htm

Joint aches
Web site:
http://www.nlm.nih.gov/medlineplus/ency/article/003261.htm

Joint stiffness
Web site:
http://www.nlm.nih.gov/medlineplus/ency/article/003261.htm

Leukemia
Web site:
http://www.nlm.nih.gov/medlineplus/ency/article/001299.htm

Macule
Web site:
http://www.nlm.nih.gov/medlineplus/ency/article/003229.htm

Malaise
Web site:
http://www.nlm.nih.gov/medlineplus/ency/article/003089.htm

Nodules
Web site:
http://www.nlm.nih.gov/medlineplus/ency/article/003230.htm

Nosebleed - symptom
Web site:
http://www.nlm.nih.gov/medlineplus/ency/article/003106.htm

Palpitations
Web site:
http://www.nlm.nih.gov/medlineplus/ency/article/003081.htm

Papule
Web site:
http://www.nlm.nih.gov/medlineplus/ency/article/003233.htm

Rales
Web site:
http://www.nlm.nih.gov/medlineplus/ency/article/003323.htm

Seizures
Web site:
http://www.nlm.nih.gov/medlineplus/ency/article/003200.htm

Shortness of breath
Web site:
http://www.nlm.nih.gov/medlineplus/ency/article/003075.htm

Skin lesion
Web site:
http://www.nlm.nih.gov/medlineplus/ency/article/003220.htm

Skin lesions
Web site:
http://www.nlm.nih.gov/medlineplus/ency/article/003220.htm

Skin rash
Web site:
http://www.nlm.nih.gov/medlineplus/ency/article/003220.htm

Skin redness
Web site:
http://www.nlm.nih.gov/medlineplus/ency/article/003220.htm

Splenomegaly
Web site:
http://www.nlm.nih.gov/medlineplus/ency/article/003276.htm

Swelling
Web site:
http://www.nlm.nih.gov/medlineplus/ency/article/003103.htm

Tearing, decreased
Web site:
http://www.nlm.nih.gov/medlineplus/ency/article/003087.htm

Visual changes
Web site:
http://www.nlm.nih.gov/medlineplus/ency/article/003029.htm

Weight loss
Web site:
http://www.nlm.nih.gov/medlineplus/ency/article/003107.htm

- **Diagnostics and Tests for Sarcoidosis**

ACE levels
Web site:
http://www.nlm.nih.gov/medlineplus/ency/article/003567.htm

Alkaline phosphatase
Web site:
http://www.nlm.nih.gov/medlineplus/ency/article/003470.htm

ALT
Web site:
http://www.nlm.nih.gov/medlineplus/ency/article/003473.htm

Biopsy
Web site:
http://www.nlm.nih.gov/medlineplus/ency/article/003416.htm

Bronchoscopy
Web site:
http://www.nlm.nih.gov/medlineplus/ency/article/003857.htm

Calcium (ionized)
Web site:
http://www.nlm.nih.gov/medlineplus/ency/article/003486.htm

Calcium; urine
Web site:
http://www.nlm.nih.gov/medlineplus/ency/article/003603.htm

CBC
Web site:
http://www.nlm.nih.gov/medlineplus/ency/article/003642.htm

Chem-20
Web site:
http://www.nlm.nih.gov/medlineplus/ency/article/003468.htm

Chem-7
Web site:
http://www.nlm.nih.gov/medlineplus/ency/article/003462.htm

Chest X-ray
Web site:
http://www.nlm.nih.gov/medlineplus/ency/article/003804.htm

CT
Web site:
http://www.nlm.nih.gov/medlineplus/ency/article/003330.htm

Gallium (Ga.) scan
Web site:
http://www.nlm.nih.gov/medlineplus/ency/article/003450.htm

Immunoelectrophoresis - serum
Web site:
http://www.nlm.nih.gov/medlineplus/ency/article/003541.htm

Kidney biopsy
Web site:
http://www.nlm.nih.gov/medlineplus/ency/article/003907.htm

Liver biopsy
Web site:
http://www.nlm.nih.gov/medlineplus/ency/article/003895.htm

Liver function tests
Web site:
http://www.nlm.nih.gov/medlineplus/ency/article/003436.htm

Lung gallium (Ga.) scan
Web site:
http://www.nlm.nih.gov/medlineplus/ency/article/003824.htm

Lymph node biopsy
Web site:
http://www.nlm.nih.gov/medlineplus/ency/article/003933.htm

Mediastinoscopy with biopsy
Web site:
http://www.nlm.nih.gov/medlineplus/ency/article/003864.htm

Nerve biopsy
Web site:
http://www.nlm.nih.gov/medlineplus/ency/article/003928.htm

Open lung biopsy
Web site:
http://www.nlm.nih.gov/medlineplus/ency/article/003861.htm

PTH
Web site:
http://www.nlm.nih.gov/medlineplus/ency/article/003690.htm

Quantitative immunoglobulins (nephelometry)
Web site:
http://www.nlm.nih.gov/medlineplus/ency/article/003545.htm

Serum calcium
Web site:
http://www.nlm.nih.gov/medlineplus/ency/article/003477.htm

Serum phosphorus
Web site:
http://www.nlm.nih.gov/medlineplus/ency/article/003478.htm

Skin lesion biopsy
Web site:
http://www.nlm.nih.gov/medlineplus/ency/article/003840.htm

X-ray
Web site:
http://www.nlm.nih.gov/medlineplus/ency/article/003337.htm

- **Background Topics for Sarcoidosis**

Acute
Web site:
http://www.nlm.nih.gov/medlineplus/ency/article/002215.htm

Analgesics
Web site:
http://www.nlm.nih.gov/medlineplus/ency/article/002123.htm

Anterior
Web site:
http://www.nlm.nih.gov/medlineplus/ency/article/002232.htm

Cardiovascular
Web site:
http://www.nlm.nih.gov/medlineplus/ency/article/002310.htm

Incidence
Web site:
http://www.nlm.nih.gov/medlineplus/ency/article/002387.htm

Peripheral
Web site:
http://www.nlm.nih.gov/medlineplus/ency/article/002273.htm

Systemic
Web site:
http://www.nlm.nih.gov/medlineplus/ency/article/002294.htm

Online Dictionary Directories

The following are additional online directories compiled by the National Library of Medicine, including a number of specialized medical dictionaries and glossaries:

- Medical Dictionaries: Medical & Biological (World Health Organization): **http://www.who.int/hlt/virtuallibrary/English/diction.htm#Medical**

- MEL-Michigan Electronic Library List of Online Health and Medical Dictionaries (Michigan Electronic Library): **http://mel.lib.mi.us/health/health-dictionaries.html**

- Patient Education: Glossaries (DMOZ Open Directory Project): **http://dmoz.org/Health/Education/Patient_Education/Glossaries/**

- Web of Online Dictionaries (Bucknell University): **http://www.yourdictionary.com/diction5.html#medicine**

SARCOIDOSIS GLOSSARY

The following is a complete glossary of terms used in this sourcebook. The definitions are derived from official public sources including the National Institutes of Health [NIH] and the European Union [EU]. After this glossary, we list a number of additional hardbound and electronic glossaries and dictionaries that you may wish to consult.

Abdomen: That portion of the body that lies between the thorax and the pelvis. [NIH]

Abscess: A localized collection of pus caused by suppuration buried in tissues, organs, or confined spaces. [EU]

Acetaminophen: Analgesic antipyretic derivative of acetanilide. It has weak anti-inflammatory properties and is used as a common analgesic, but may cause liver, blood cell, and kidney damage. [NIH]

Acne: An inflammatory disease of the pilosebaceous unit, the specific type usually being indicated by a modifying term; frequently used alone to designate common acne, or acne vulgaris. [EU]

Algorithms: A procedure consisting of a sequence of algebraic formulas and/or logical steps to calculate or determine a given task. [NIH]

Alkaline Phosphatase: An enzyme that catalyzes the conversion of an orthophosphoric monoester and water to an alcohol and orthophosphate. EC 3.1.3.1. [NIH]

Analgesic: An agent that alleviates pain without causing loss of consciousness. [EU]

Anaphylaxis: An acute hypersensitivity reaction due to exposure to a previously encountered antigen. The reaction may include rapidly progressing urticaria, respiratory distress, vascular collapse, systemic shock, and death. [NIH]

Anemia: A reduction in the number of circulating erythrocytes or in the quantity of hemoglobin. [NIH]

Anergy: Absence of immune response to particular substances. [NIH]

Anesthesia: A state characterized by loss of feeling or sensation. This depression of nerve function is usually the result of pharmacologic action and is induced to allow performance of surgery or other painful procedures. [NIH]

Angioedema: A vascular reaction involving the deep dermis or subcutaneous or submucal tissues, representing localized edema caused by dilatation and increased permeability of the capillaries, and characterized by development of giant wheals. [EU]

Ankle: That part of the lower limb directly above the foot. [NIH]

Antibiotic: A drug that kills or inhibits the growth of bacteria. [NIH]

Antibodies: Specific proteins produced by the body's immune system that bind with foreign proteins (antigens). [NIH]

Antibody: An immunoglobulin molecule that has a specific amino acid sequence by virtue of which it interacts only with the antigen that induced its synthesis in cells of the lymphoid series (especially plasma cells), or with antigen closely related to it. Antibodies are classified according to their ode of action as agglutinins, bacteriolysins, haemolysins, opsonins, precipitins, etc. [EU]

Antigen: Any substance which is capable, under appropriate conditions, of inducing a specific immune response and of reacting with the products of that response, that is, with specific antibody or specifically sensitized T-lymphocytes, or both. Antigens may be soluble substances, such as toxins and foreign proteins, or particulate, such as bacteria and tissue cells; however, only the portion of the protein or polysaccharide molecule known as the antigenic determinant (q.v.) combines with antibody or a specific receptor on a lymphocyte. Abbreviated Ag. [EU]

Antimicrobial: Killing microorganisms, or suppressing their multiplication or growth. [EU]

Antineoplastic: Inhibiting or preventing the development of neoplasms, checking the maturation and proliferation of malignant cells. [EU]

Anxiety: The unpleasant emotional state consisting of psychophysiological responses to anticipation of unreal or imagined danger, ostensibly resulting from unrecognized intrapsychic conflict. Physiological concomitants include increased heart rate, altered respiration rate, sweating, trembling, weakness, and fatigue; psychological concomitants include feelings of impending danger, powerlessness, apprehension, and tension. [EU]

Apnea: A transient absence of spontaneous respiration. [NIH]

Aqueous: Watery; prepared with water. [EU]

Arrhythmia: An irregular heartbeat. [NIH]

Arteries: The vessels carrying blood away from the heart. [NIH]

Arteriography: Roentgenography of arteries after injection of radiopacque material into the blood stream. [EU]

Arthralgia: Pain in a joint. [EU]

Arthropathy: Any joint disease. [EU]

Aspergillus: A genus of mitosporic fungi containing about 100 species and eleven different teleomorphs in the family Trichocomaceae. [NIH]

Aspiration: The act of inhaling. [EU]

Assay: Determination of the amount of a particular constituent of a mixture, or of the biological or pharmacological potency of a drug. [EU]

Asymptomatic: Showing or causing no symptoms. [EU]

Atrophy: A wasting away; a diminution in the size of a cell, tissue, organ, or part. [EU]

Audiology: The study of hearing and hearing impairment. [NIH]

Auscultation: The act of listening for sounds within the body, chiefly for ascertaining the condition of the lungs, heart, pleura, abdomen and other organs, and for the detection of pregnancy. [EU]

Autoimmunity: Process whereby the immune system reacts against the body's own tissues. Autoimmunity may produce or be caused by autoimmune diseases. [NIH]

Barotrauma: Injury following pressure changes; includes injury to the eustachian tube, ear drum, lung and stomach. [NIH]

Benign: Not malignant; not recurrent; favourable for recovery. [EU]

Benzodiazepines: A two-ring heterocyclic compound consisting of a benzene ring fused to a diazepine ring. Permitted is any degree of hydrogenation, any substituents and any H-isomer. [NIH]

Berylliosis: A lung disease resulting from exposure to beryllium metal. [NIH]

Beryllium: Beryllium. An element with the atomic symbol Be, atomic number 4, and atomic weight 9.01218. Short exposure to this element can lead to a type of poisoning known as berylliosis. [NIH]

Bilateral: Having two sides, or pertaining to both sides. [EU]

Biliary: Pertaining to the bile, to the bile ducts, or to the gallbladder. [EU]

Biochemical: Relating to biochemistry; characterized by, produced by, or involving chemical reactions in living organisms. [EU]

Biopsy: The removal and examination, usually microscopic, of tissue from the living body, performed to establish precise diagnosis. [EU]

Blindness: The inability to see or the loss or absence of perception of visual stimuli. This condition may be the result of eye diseases; optic nerve diseases; optic chiasm diseases; or brain diseases affecting the visual pathways or occipital lobe. [NIH]

Bronchiectasis: Chronic dilatation of the bronchi marked by fetid breath and paroxysmal coughing, with the expectoration of mucopurulent matter. It may effect the tube uniformly (cylindric b.), or occur in irregular pockets (sacculated b.) or the dilated tubes may have terminal bulbous enlargements (fusiform b.). [EU]

Bronchitis: Inflammation of one or more bronchi. [EU]

Bronchoscope: A long, narrow tube with a light at the end that is used by the doctor for direct observation of the airways, as well as for suction of tissue and other materials. [NIH]

Bronchoscopy: A technique for visualizing the interior of bronchi and instilling or removing fluid or tissue samples by passing a lighted tube (bronchoscope) through the nose or mouth into the bronchi. [NIH]

Buccal: Pertaining to or directed toward the cheek. In dental anatomy, used to refer to the buccal surface of a tooth. [EU]

Calcitonin: A peptide hormone that lowers calcium concentration in the blood. In humans, it is released by thyroid cells and acts to decrease the formation and absorptive activity of osteoclasts. Its role in regulating plasma calcium is much greater in children and in certain diseases than in normal adults. [NIH]

Carbohydrates: A nutrient that supplies 4 calories/gram. They may be simple or complex. Simple carbohydrates are called sugars, and complex carbohydrates are called starch and fiber (cellulose). An organic compound—containing carbon, hydrogen, and oxygen—that is formed by photosynthesis in plants. Carbohydrates are heat producing and are classified as monosaccharides, disaccharides, or polysaccharides. [NIH]

Carcinoma: A malignant new growth made up of epithelial cells tending to infiltrate the surrounding tissues and give rise to metastases. [EU]

Cardiac: Pertaining to the heart. [EU]

Cardiovascular: Pertaining to the heart and blood vessels. [EU]

Cataract: An opacity, partial or complete, of one or both eyes, on or in the lens or capsule, especially an opacity impairing vision or causing blindness. The many kinds of cataract are classified by their morphology (size, shape, location) or etiology (cause and time of occurrence). [EU]

Caustic: An escharotic or corrosive agent. Called also cauterant. [EU]

Cell: Basic subunit of every living organism; the simplest unit that can exist as an independent living system. [NIH]

Chancre: The primary sore of syphilis, a painless indurated, eroded papule, occurring at the site of entry of the infection. [NIH]

Cheilitis: Inflammation of the lips. It is of various etiologies and degrees of pathology. [NIH]

Chemotherapy: The treatment of disease by means of chemicals that have a specific toxic effect upon the disease - producing microorganisms or that selectively destroy cancerous tissue. [EU]

Chloroquine: The prototypical antimalarial agent with a mechanism that is not well understood. It has also been used to treat rheumatoid arthritis, systemic lupus erythematosus, and in the systemic therapy of amebic liver abscesses. [NIH]

Cholangitis: Inflammation of a bile duct. [EU]

Cholecystitis: Inflammation of the gallbladder, caused primarily by gallstones. Gallbladder disease occurs most often in obese women older than 40 years of age. [NIH]

Cholesterol: A soft, waxy substance manufactured by the body and used in the production of hormones, bile acid, and vitamin D and present in all parts of the body, including the nervous system, muscle, skin, liver, intestines, and heart. Blood cholesterol circulates in the bloodstream. Dietary cholesterol is found in foods of animal origin. [NIH]

Chromosomal: Pertaining to chromosomes. [EU]

Chronic: Of long duration; frequently recurring. [NIH]

Cirrhosis: Liver disease characterized pathologically by loss of the normal microscopic lobular architecture, with fibrosis and nodular regeneration. The term is sometimes used to refer to chronic interstitial inflammation of any organ. [EU]

Cisplatin: An inorganic and water-soluble platinum complex. After undergoing hydrolysis, it reacts with DNA to produce both intra and interstrand crosslinks. These crosslinks appear to impair replication and transcription of DNA. The cytotoxicity of cisplatin correlates with cellular arrest in the G2 phase of the cell cycle. [NIH]

Cochlear: Of or pertaining to the cochlea. [EU]

Colitis: Inflammation of the colon. [EU]

Collagen: The protein substance of the white fibres (collagenous fibres) of skin, tendon, bone, cartilage, and all other connective tissue; composed of molecules of tropocollagen (q.v.), it is converted into gelatin by boiling. collagenous pertaining to collagen; forming or producing collagen. [EU]

Cornea: The transparent structure forming the anterior part of the fibrous tunic of the eye. It consists of five layers : (1) the anterior corneal epithelium, continuous with that of the conjunctiva, (2) the anterior limiting layer (Bowman's membrane), (3) the substantia propria, or stroma, (4) the posterior limiting layer (Descemet's membrane), and (5) the endothelium of the anterior chamber, called also keratoderma. [EU]

Corticosteroids: Drugs that mimic the action of a group of hormones produced by adrenal glands; they are anti-inflammatory and act as bronchodilators. [NIH]

Cryoglobulinemia: A condition characterized by the presence of abnormal or abnormal quantities of cryoglobulins in the blood. They are precipitated into the microvasculature on exposure to cold and cause restricted blood flow in exposed areas. [NIH]

Cryptococcosis: Infection with a fungus of the species cryptococcus neoformans. [NIH]

Cryptococcus: A mitosporic Tremellales fungal genus whose species usually have a capsule and do not form pseudomycellium. Teleomorphs include Filobasidiella and Fidobasidium. [NIH]

Cutaneous: Pertaining to the skin; dermal; dermic. [EU]

Cyclophosphamide: Precursor of an alkylating nitrogen mustard antineoplastic and immunosuppressive agent that must be activated in the liver to form the active aldophosphamide. It is used in the treatment of lymphomas, leukemias, etc. Its side effect, alopecia, has been made use of in defleecing sheep. Cyclophosphamide may also cause sterility, birth defects, mutations, and cancer. [NIH]

Cyst: Any closed cavity or sac; normal or abnormal, lined by epithelium, and especially one that contains a liquid or semisolid material. [EU]

Cytokines: Non-antibody proteins secreted by inflammatory leukocytes and some non-leukocytic cells, that act as intercellular mediators. They differ from classical hormones in that they are produced by a number of tissue or cell types rather than by specialized glands. They generally act locally in a paracrine or autocrine rather than endocrine manner. [NIH]

Cytomegalovirus: A genus of the family herpesviridae, subfamily betaherpesvirinae, infecting the salivary glands, liver, spleen, lungs, eyes, and other organs, in which they produce characteristically enlarged cells with intranuclear inclusions. Infection with Cytomegalovirus is also seen as an opportunistic infection in AIDS. [NIH]

Cytotoxic: Pertaining to or exhibiting cytotoxicity. [EU]

Degenerative: Undergoing degeneration : tending to degenerate; having the character of or involving degeneration; causing or tending to cause degeneration. [EU]

Dermatology: A medical specialty concerned with the skin, its structure, functions, diseases, and treatment. [NIH]

Dermatosis: Any skin disease, especially one not characterized by inflammation. [EU]

Diarrhea: Passage of excessively liquid or excessively frequent stools. [NIH]

Digestion: The process of breakdown of food for metabolism and use by the body. [NIH]

Diverticulitis: Inflammation of a diverticulum, especially inflammation related to colonic diverticula, which may undergo perforation with abscess formation. Sometimes called left-sided or L-sides appendicitis. [EU]

Dysplasia: Abnormal development or growth. [NIH]

Dyspnea: Shortness of breath; difficult or labored breathing. [NIH]

Dystrophy: Any disorder arising from defective or faulty nutrition, especially the muscular dystrophies. [EU]

Efficacy: The extent to which a specific intervention, procedure, regimen, or service produces a beneficial result under ideal conditions. Ideally, the determination of efficacy is based on the results of a randomized control trial. [NIH]

Electrolyte: A substance that dissociates into ions when fused or in solution, and thus becomes capable of conducting electricity; an ionic solute. [EU]

Emphysema: Chronic lung disease in which there is permanent destruction of alveoli. [NIH]

Endogenous: Developing or originating within the organisms or arising from causes within the organism. [EU]

Enzyme: Substance, made by living cells, that causes specific chemical changes. [NIH]

Epidemiological: Relating to, or involving epidemiology. [EU]

Erythema: A name applied to redness of the skin produced by congestion of the capillaries, which may result from a variety of causes, the etiology or a specific type of lesion often being indicated by a modifying term. [EU]

Erythrocytes: Red blood cells. Mature erythrocytes are non-nucleated, biconcave disks containing hemoglobin whose function is to transport oxygen. [NIH]

Erythromycin: A bacteriostatic antibiotic substance produced by Streptomyces erythreus. Erythromycin A is considered its major active component. In sensitive organisms, it inhibits protein synthesis by binding to 50S ribosomal subunits. This binding process inhibits peptidyl transferase activity and interferes with translocation of amino acids during translation and assembly of proteins. [NIH]

Estradiol: The most potent mammalian estrogenic hormone. It is produced in the ovary, placenta, testis, and possibly the adrenal cortex. [NIH]

Exogenous: Developed or originating outside the organism, as exogenous disease. [EU]

Fatigue: The state of weariness following a period of exertion, mental or physical, characterized by a decreased capacity for work and reduced efficiency to respond to stimuli. [NIH]

Fetus: Unborn offspring from 7 or 8 weeks after conception until birth. [NIH]

Fibroblasts: Connective tissue cells which secrete an extracellular matrix rich in collagen and other macromolecules. [NIH]

Fibrosis: Process by which inflamed tissue becomes scarred. [NIH]

Fluorouracil: A pyrimidine analog that acts as an antineoplastic antimetabolite and also has immunosuppressant. It interferes with DNA synthesis by blocking the thymidylate synthetase conversion of deoxyuridylic acid to thymidylic acid. [NIH]

Gallium: A rare, metallic element designated by the symbol, Ga, atomic number 31, and atomic weight 69.72. [NIH]

Gastritis: Inflammation of the stomach. [EU]

Gastrointestinal: Pertaining to or communicating with the stomach and intestine, as a gastrointestinal fistula. [EU]

Genitourinary: Pertaining to the genital and urinary organs; urogenital; urinosexual. [EU]

Gingivitis: Inflammation of the gingivae. Gingivitis associated with bony changes is referred to as periodontitis. Called also oulitis and ulitis. [EU]

Glomerular: Pertaining to or of the nature of a glomerulus, especially a renal glomerulus. [EU]

Glomerulonephritis: A variety of nephritis characterized by inflammation of the capillary loops in the glomeruli of the kidney. It occurs in acute, subacute, and chronic forms and may be secondary to haemolytic streptococcal infection. Evidence also supports possible immune or autoimmune mechanisms. [EU]

Gluten: The protein of wheat and other grains which gives to the dough its tough elastic character. [EU]

Gout: Hereditary metabolic disorder characterized by recurrent acute arthritis, hyperuricemia and deposition of sodium urate in and around the joints, sometimes with formation of uric acid calculi. [NIH]

Granulomas: Small lumps in tissues caused by inflammation. [NIH]

Heartbeat: One complete contraction of the heart. [NIH]

Hematology: A subspecialty of internal medicine concerned with morphology, physiology, and pathology of the blood and blood-forming tissues. [NIH]

Hemoptysis: Coughing up blood or blood-stained sputum. [NIH]

Hepatic: Pertaining to the liver. [EU]

Hepatitis: Inflammation of the liver. [EU]

Hepatomegaly: Enlargement of the liver. [EU]

Heredity: 1. the genetic transmission of a particular quality or trait from parent to offspring. 2. the genetic constitution of an individual. [EU]

Herpes: Any inflammatory skin disease caused by a herpesvirus and characterized by the formation of clusters of small vesicles. When used alone, the term may refer to herpes simplex or to herpes zoster. [EU]

Histamine: 1H-Imidazole-4-ethanamine. A depressor amine derived by enzymatic decarboxylation of histidine. It is a powerful stimulant of gastric secretion, a constrictor of bronchial smooth muscle, a vasodilator, and also a centrally acting neurotransmitter. [NIH]

Histiocytosis: General term for the abnormal appearance of histiocytes in the blood. Based on the pathological features of the cells involved rather than on clinical findings, the histiocytic diseases are subdivided into three groups: Histiocytosis, Langerhans Cell; Histiocytosis, Non-Langerhans Cell; And Histiocytic Disorders, Malignant. [NIH]

Histocompatibility: The degree of antigenic similarity between the tissues of different individuals, which determines the acceptance or rejection of allografts. [NIH]

Homeostasis: A tendency to stability in the normal body states (internal environment) of the organism. It is achieved by a system of control mechanisms activated by negative feedback; e.g. a high level of carbon dioxide in extracellular fluid triggers increased pulmonary ventilation, which in turn causes a decrease in carbon dioxide concentration. [EU]

Hormonal: Pertaining to or of the nature of a hormone. [EU]

Humoral: Of, relating to, proceeding from, or involving a bodily humour - now often used of endocrine factors as opposed to neural or somatic. [EU]

Hypercalcemia: Abnormally high level of calcium in the blood. [NIH]

Hyperlipoproteinemia: Metabolic disease characterized by elevated plasma cholesterol and/or triglyceride levels. The inherited form is attributed to a single gene mechanism. [NIH]

Hyperostosis: Hypertrophy of bone; exostosis. [EU]

Hyperpigmentation: Excessive pigmentation of the skin, usually as a result of increased melanization of the epidermis rather than as a result of an increased number of melanocytes. Etiology is varied and the condition may arise from exposure to light, chemicals or other substances, or from a primary metabolic imbalance. [NIH]

Hypersensitivity: A state of altered reactivity in which the body reacts with an exaggerated immune response to a foreign substance. Hypersensitivity reactions are classified as immediate or delayed, types I and IV, respectively, in the Gell and Coombs classification (q.v.) of immune responses. [EU]

Hypertension: High blood pressure (i.e., abnormally high blood pressure tension involving systolic and/or diastolic levels). The Sixth Report of the Joint National Committee on Prevention, Detection, Evaluation, and Treatment of High Blood Pressure defines hypertension as a systolic blood pressure of 140 mm Hg or greater, a diastolic blood pressure of 90 mm Hg or greater, or taking hypertensive medication. The cause may be adrenal, benign, essential, Goldblatt's, idiopathic, malignant PATE, portal, postpartum, primary, pulmonary, renal or renovascular. [NIH]

Hyperthermia: Abnormally high body temperature, especially that induced for therapeutic purposes. [EU]

Hyperthyroidism: 1. excessive functional activity of the thyroid gland. 2. the abnormal condition resulting from hyperthyroidism marked by increased metabolic rate, enlargement of the thyroid gland, rapid heart rate, high blood pressure, and various secondary symptoms. [EU]

Hypothyroidism: Deficiency of thyroid activity. In adults, it is most common in women and is characterized by decrease in basal metabolic rate, tiredness and lethargy, sensitivity to cold, and menstrual disturbances. If untreated, it progresses to full-blown myxoedema. In infants, severe hypothyroidism leads to cretinism. In juveniles, the manifestations are intermediate, with less severe mental and developmental retardation and only mild symptoms of the adult form. When due to pituitary deficiency of thyrotropin secretion it is called secondary hypothyroidism. [EU]

Iatrogenic: Resulting from the activity of physicians. Originally applied to disorders induced in the patient by autosuggestion based on the physician's examination, manner, or discussion, the term is now applied to any adverse condition in a patient occurring as the result of treatment by a physician or surgeon, especially to infections acquired by the patient during the course of treatment. [EU]

Idiopathic: Results from an unknown cause. [NIH]

Immunotherapy: Manipulation of the host's immune system in treatment of disease. It includes both active and passive immunization as well as immunosuppressive therapy to prevent graft rejection. [NIH]

Impetigo: A common superficial bacterial infection caused by staphylococcus aureus or group A beta-hemolytic streptococci. Characteristics include pustular lesions that rupture and discharge a thin, amber-colored fluid that dries and forms a crust. This condition is commonly located on the face, especially about the mouth and nose. [NIH]

Infiltration: The diffusion or accumulation in a tissue or cells of substances not normal to it or in amounts of the normal. Also, the material so accumulated. [EU]

Inflammation: Response of the body tissues to injury; typical signs are swelling, redness, and pain. [NIH]

Inhalation: The drawing of air or other substances into the lungs. [EU]

Insulin: A protein hormone secreted by beta cells of the pancreas. Insulin plays a major role in the regulation of glucose metabolism, generally promoting the cellular utilization of glucose. It is also an important regulator of protein and lipid metabolism. Insulin is used as a drug to control insulin-dependent diabetes mellitus. [NIH]

Intermittent: Occurring at separated intervals; having periods of cessation of activity. [EU]

Interstitial: Pertaining to or situated between parts or in the interspaces of a tissue. [EU]

Invasive: 1. having the quality of invasiveness. 2. involving puncture or incision of the skin or insertion of an instrument or foreign material into the body; said of diagnostic techniques. [EU]

Iodine: A nonmetallic element of the halogen group that is represented by the atomic symbol I, atomic number 53, and atomic weight of 126.90. It is a nutritionally essential element, especially important in thyroid hormone synthesis. In solution, it has anti-infective properties and is used topically. [NIH]

Iridocyclitis: Inflammation of the iris and of the ciliary body; anterior uveitis. [EU]

Isotretinoin: A topical dermatologic agent that is used in the treatment of acne vulgaris and several other skin diseases. The drug has teratogenic and other adverse effects. [NIH]

Keloid: A sharply elevated, irregularly- shaped, progressively enlarging scar due to the formation of excessive amounts of collagen in the corium during connective tissue repair. [EU]

Labyrinthitis: Inflammation of the inner ear. [NIH]

Lavage: To wash the interior of a body organ. [NIH]

Legionellosis: Infections with bacteria of the genus legionella. [NIH]

Leprosy: A chronic granulomatous infection caused by mycobacterium leprae. The granulomatous lesions are manifested in the skin, the mucous membranes, and the peripheral nerves. Two polar or principal types are lepromatous and tuberculoid. [NIH]

Lesion: Any pathological or traumatic discontinuity of tissue or loss of function of a part. [EU]

Leucine: An essential branched-chain amino acid important for hemoglobin formation. [NIH]

LH: A small glycoprotein hormone secreted by the anterior pituitary. LH plays an important role in controlling ovulation and in controlling secretion of hormones by the ovaries and testes. [NIH]

Lipodystrophy: 1. any disturbance of fat metabolism. 2. a group of conditions due to defective metabolism of fat, resulting in the absence of subcutaneous fat, which may be congenital or acquired and partial or total. Called also lipoatrophy and lipodystrophia. [EU]

Liquifilm: A thin liquid layer of coating. [EU]

Lubrication: The application of a substance to diminish friction between two surfaces. It may refer to oils, greases, and similar substances for the lubrication of medical equipment but it can be used for the application of substances to tissue to reduce friction, such as lotions for skin and vaginal lubricants. [NIH]

Lumbar: Pertaining to the loins, the part of the back between the thorax and the pelvis. [EU]

Lupus: A form of cutaneous tuberculosis. It is seen predominantly in women and typically involves the nasal, buccal, and conjunctival mucosa. [NIH]

Lymph: A transparent, slightly yellow liquid found in the lymphatic vessels. Lymph is collected from tissue fluids throughout the body and returned to the blood via the lymphatic system. [NIH]

Lymphadenopathy: Disease of the lymph nodes. [EU]

Lymphocytic: Pertaining to, characterized by, or of the nature of lymphocytes. [EU]

Lymphoma: Cancer of the lymph nodes. [NIH]

Lymphopenia: Reduction in the number of lymphocytes. [NIH]

Maculopapular: Both macular and papular, as an eruption consisting of both macules and papules; sometimes erroneously used to designate a papule that is only slightly elevated. [EU]

Malaise: A vague feeling of bodily discomfort. [EU]

Masticatory: 1. subserving or pertaining to mastication; affecting the muscles of mastication. 2. a remedy to be chewed but not swallowed. [EU]

Mediator: An object or substance by which something is mediated, such as (1) a structure of the nervous system that transmits impulses eliciting a specific response; (2) a chemical substance (transmitter substance) that induces activity in an excitable tissue, such as nerve or muscle; or (3) a substance released from cells as the result of the interaction of antigen with antibody or by the action of antigen with a sensitized lymphocyte. [EU]

Membrane: Thin, flexible film of proteins and lipids that encloses the contents of a cell; it controls the substances that go into and come out of the cell. Also, a thin layer of tissue that covers the surface or lines the cavity of an organ. [NIH]

Meningitis: Inflammation of the meninges. When it affects the dura mater, the disease is termed pachymeningitis; when the arachnoid and pia mater are involved, it is called leptomeningitis, or meningitis proper. [EU]

Methimazole: A thioureylene antithyroid agent that inhibits the formation of thyroid hormones by interfering with the incorporation of iodine into tyrosyl residues of thyroglobulin. This is done by interfering with the oxidation of iodide ion and iodotyrosyl groups through inhibition of the peroxidase enzyme. [NIH]

Methotrexate: An antineoplastic antimetabolite with immunosuppressant properties. It is an inhibitor of dihydrofolate reductase and prevents the formation of tetrahydrofolate, necessary for synthesis of thymidylate, an essential component of DNA. [NIH]

Microbiology: The study of microorganisms such as fungi, bacteria, algae, archaea, and viruses. [NIH]

Molecular: Of, pertaining to, or composed of molecules : a very small mass of matter. [EU]

Monocytes: Large, phagocytic mononuclear leukocytes produced in the vertebrate bone marrow and released into the blood; contain a large, oval or somewhat indented nucleus surrounded by voluminous cytoplasm and numerous organelles. [NIH]

Mononucleosis: The presence of an abnormally large number of mononuclear leucocytes (monocytes) in the blood. The term is often used alone to refer to infectious mononucleosis. [EU]

Mucosa: A mucous membrane, or tunica mucosa. [EU]

Mucus: A thick fluid produced by the lining of some organs of the body. [NIH]

Mycobacterium: An organism of the genus Mycobacterium. [EU]

Mycoplasma: A genus of gram-negative, facultatively anaerobic bacteria bounded by a plasma membrane only. Its organisms are parasites and pathogens, found on the mucous membranes of humans, animals, and birds. [NIH]

Myeloma: A tumour composed of cells of the type normally found in the bone marrow. [EU]

Myocarditis: Inflammation of the myocardium; inflammation of the muscular walls of the heart. [EU]

Nasal: Pertaining to the nose. [EU]

Nausea: An unpleasant sensation, vaguely referred to the epigastrium and abdomen, and often culminating in vomiting. [EU]

Necrosis: The sum of the morphological changes indicative of cell death and caused by the progressive degradative action of enzymes; it may affect groups of cells or part of a structure or an organ. [EU]

Neonatal: Pertaining to the first four weeks after birth. [EU]

Neoplasms: New abnormal growth of tissue. Malignant neoplasms show a greater degree of anaplasia and have the properties of invasion and metastasis, compared to benign neoplasms. [NIH]

Neoplastic: Pertaining to or like a neoplasm (= any new and abnormal growth); pertaining to neoplasia (= the formation of a neoplasm). [EU]

Nephrology: A subspecialty of internal medicine concerned with the anatomy, physiology, and pathology of the kidney. [NIH]

Nephrons: The functional units of the kidney, consisting of the glomerulus and the attached tubule. [NIH]

Nephropathy: Disease of the kidneys. [EU]

Neurology: A medical specialty concerned with the study of the structures, functions, and diseases of the nervous system. [NIH]

Nevirapine: A potent, non-nucleoside reverse transcriptase inhibitor used in combination with nucleoside analogues for treatment of HIV infection and AIDS. [NIH]

Niacin: Water-soluble vitamin of the B complex occurring in various animal and plant tissues. Required by the body for the formation of coenzymes NAD and NADP. Has pellagra-curative, vasodilating, and antilipemic properties. [NIH]

Nitrogen: An element with the atomic symbol N, atomic number 7, and atomic weight 14. Nitrogen exists as a diatomic gas and makes up about 78% of the earth's atmosphere by volume. It is a constituent of proteins and nucleic acids and found in all living cells. [NIH]

Ophthalmology: A surgical specialty concerned with the structure and function of the eye and the medical and surgical treatment of its defects and diseases. [NIH]

Osteoarthritis: Noninflammatory degenerative joint disease occurring chiefly in older persons, characterized by degeneration of the articular cartilage, hypertrophy of bone at the margins, and changes in the synovial membrane. It is accompanied by pain and stiffness. [NIH]

Osteodystrophy: Defective bone formation. [EU]

Osteogenesis: The histogenesis of bone including ossification. It occurs continuously but particularly in the embryo and child and during fracture repair. [NIH]

Osteonecrosis: Death of a bone or part of a bone, either atraumatic or posttraumatic. [NIH]

Osteopetrosis: Excessive formation of dense trabecular bone leading to pathological fractures, osteitis, splenomegaly with infarct, anemia, and extramedullary hemopoiesis. [NIH]

Osteoporosis: Reduction in the amount of bone mass, leading to fractures after minimal trauma. [EU]

Otolaryngology: A surgical specialty concerned with the study and treatment of disorders of the ear, nose, and throat. [NIH]

Otorhinolaryngology: That branch of medicine concerned with medical and surgical treatment of the head and neck, including the ears, nose and throat. [EU]

Otosclerosis: A pathological condition of the bony labyrinth of the ear, in which there is formation of spongy bone (otospongiosis), especially in front of and posterior to the footplate of the stapes; it may cause bony ankylosis of the stapes, resulting in conductive hearing loss. Cochlear otosclerosis may also develop, resulting in sensorineural hearing loss. [EU]

Overweight: An excess of body weight but not necessarily body fat; a body mass index of 25 to 29.9 kg/m2. [NIH]

Pacemaker: An object or substance that influences the rate at which a certain phenomenon occurs; often used alone to indicate the natural cardiac pacemaker or an artificial cardiac pacemaker. In biochemistry, a substance whose rate of reaction sets the pace for a series of interrelated reactions. [EU]

Palliative: 1. affording relief, but not cure. 2. an alleviating medicine. [EU]

Palpitation: The sensation of rapid heartbeats. [NIH]

Pancreas: A mixed exocrine and endocrine gland situated transversely across the posterior abdominal wall in the epigastric and hypochondriac regions. The endocrine portion is comprised of the islets of langerhans, while the exocrine portion is a compound acinar gland that secretes digestive enzymes. [NIH]

Panniculitis: An inflammatory reaction of the subcutaneous fat, which may involve the connective tissue septa between the fat lobes, the septa lobules and vessels, or the fat lobules, characterized by the development of single or multiple cutaneous nodules. [EU]

Papule: A small circumscribed, superficial, solid elevation of the skin. [EU]

Paralysis: Loss or impairment of motor function in a part due to lesion of the neural or muscular mechanism; also by analogy, impairment of sensory function (sensory paralysis). In addition to the types named below, paralysis is further distinguished as traumatic, syphilitic, toxic, etc., according to its cause; or as obturator, ulnar, etc., according to the nerve part, or muscle specially affected. [EU]

Parotitis: Inflammation of the parotid gland. Called also parotiditis. [EU]

Pathogenesis: The cellular events and reactions that occur in the development of disease. [NIH]

Pathologic: 1. indicative of or caused by a morbid condition. 2. pertaining to pathology (= branch of medicine that treats the essential nature of the disease, especially the structural and functional changes in tissues and organs of the body caused by the disease). [EU]

Penicillamine: 3-Mercapto-D-valine. The most characteristic degradation product of the penicillin antibiotics. It is used as an antirheumatic and as a chelating agent in Wilson's disease. [NIH]

Pentoxifylline: A methylxanthine derivative that inhibits phosphodiesterase and affects blood rheology. It improves blood flow by increasing erythrocyte and leukocyte flexibility. It also inhibits platelet aggregation. Pentoxifylline modulates immunologic activity by stimulating cytokine production. [NIH]

Perineal: Pertaining to the perineum. [EU]

PFT: Pulmonary function test. [NIH]

Phenotype: The entire physical, biochemical, and physiological makeup of an individual as determined by his or her genes and by the environment in the broad sense. [NIH]

Physiologic: Normal; not pathologic; characteristic of or conforming to the normal functioning or state of the body or a tissue or organ; physiological. [EU]

Pilocarpine: A slowly hydrolyzed muscarinic agonist with no nicotinic effects. Pilocarpine is used as a miotic and in the treatment of glaucoma. [NIH]

Pneumonia: Inflammation of the lungs. [NIH]

Pneumonitis: A disease caused by inhaling a wide variety of substances such as dusts and molds. Also called "farmer's disease". [NIH]

Podophyllum: A genus of poisonous American herbs, family Berberidaceae. The roots yield podophyllotoxins and other pharmacologically important agents. The plant was formerly used as a cholagogue and cathartic. It is different from the European mandrake, mandragora. [NIH]

Porphyria: A pathological state in man and some lower animals that is often due to genetic factors, is characterized by abnormalities of porphyrin metabolism, and results in the excretion of large quantities of porphyrins in the urine and in extreme sensitivity to light. [EU]

Potassium: An element that is in the alkali group of metals. It has an atomic symbol K, atomic number 19, and atomic weight 39.10. It is the chief cation in the intracellular fluid of muscle and other cells. Potassium ion is a strong electrolyte and it plays a significant role in the regulation of fluid volume and maintenance of the water-electrolyte balance. [NIH]

Predisposition: A latent susceptibility to disease which may be activated under certain conditions, as by stress. [EU]

Prednisone: A synthetic anti-inflammatory glucocorticoid derived from cortisone. It is biologically inert and converted to prednisolone in the liver. [NIH]

Presbycusis: Progressive bilateral loss of hearing that occurs in the aged. Syn: senile deafness. [NIH]

Proctitis: Inflammation of the rectum. [EU]

Proteins: Polymers of amino acids linked by peptide bonds. The specific sequence of amino acids determines the shape and function of the protein. [NIH]

Psoriasis: A common genetically determined, chronic, inflammatory skin disease characterized by rounded erythematous, dry, scaling patches. The lesions have a predilection for nails, scalp, genitalia, extensor surfaces, and the lumbosacral region. Accelerated epidermopoiesis is considered to be the fundamental pathologic feature in psoriasis. [NIH]

Pulmonary: Relating to the lungs. [NIH]

Pyoderma: Any purulent skin disease. Called also pyodermia. [EU]

Pyogenic: Producing pus; pyopoietic (= liquid inflammation product made up of cells and a thin fluid called liquor puris). [EU]

Radioactivity: The quality of emitting or the emission of corpuscular or electromagnetic radiations consequent to nuclear disintegration, a natural property of all chemical elements of atomic number above 83, and possible of induction in all other known elements. [EU]

Radiography: The making of film records (radiographs) of internal structures of the body by passage of x-rays or gamma rays through the body to act on specially sensitized film. [EU]

Radiology: A specialty concerned with the use of x-ray and other forms of radiant energy in the diagnosis and treatment of disease. [NIH]

Radiotherapy: The treatment of disease by ionizing radiation. [EU]

Receptor: 1. a molecular structure within a cell or on the surface characterized by (1) selective binding of a specific substance and (2) a specific physiologic effect that accompanies the binding, e.g., cell-surface receptors for peptide hormones, neurotransmitters, antigens, complement fragments, and immunoglobulins and cytoplasmic receptors for steroid hormones. 2. a sensory nerve terminal that responds to stimuli of various kinds. [EU]

Rectal: Pertaining to the rectum (= distal portion of the large intestine). [EU]

Reflux: A backward or return flow. [EU]

Remission: A diminution or abatement of the symptoms of a disease; also the period during which such diminution occurs. [EU]

Renovascular: Of or pertaining to the blood vessels of the kidneys. [EU]

Retina: The inner layer of tissue at the back of the eye that is sensitive to light. [NIH]

Rheumatoid: Resembling rheumatism. [EU]

Rheumatology: A subspecialty of internal medicine concerned with the study of inflammatory or degenerative processes and metabolic derangement of connective tissue structures which pertain to a variety of musculoskeletal disorders, such as arthritis. [NIH]

Rhinitis: Inflammation of the mucous membrane of the nose. [EU]

Riboflavin: Nutritional factor found in milk, eggs, malted barley, liver, kidney, heart, and leafy vegetables. The richest natural source is yeast. It occurs in the free form only in the retina of the eye, in whey, and in urine; its principal forms in tissues and cells are as FMN and FAD. [NIH]

Rubella: An acute, usually benign, infectious disease caused by a togavirus and most often affecting children and nonimmune young adults, in which the virus enters the respiratory tract via droplet nuclei and spreads to the lymphatic system. It is characterized by a slight cold, sore throat, and fever, followed by enlargement of the postauricular, suboccipital, and cervical lymph nodes, and the appearances of a fine pink rash that begins on the head and spreads to become generalized. Called also German measles, roetln, röteln, and three-day measles, and rubeola in French and Spanish. [EU]

Sarcoidosis: An idiopathic systemic inflammatory granulomatous disorder comprised of epithelioid and multinucleated giant cells with little necrosis. It usually invades the lungs with fibrosis and may also involve lymph nodes, skin, liver, spleen, eyes, phalangeal bones, and parotid glands. [NIH]

Sclera: Outer coat of the eyeball. [NIH]

Sclerosis: A induration, or hardening; especially hardening of a part from inflammation and in diseases of the interstitial substance. The term is used chiefly for such a hardening of the nervous system due to hyperplasia of the connective tissue or to designate hardening of the blood vessels. [EU]

Sedimentation: The act of causing the deposit of sediment, especially by the use of a centrifugal machine. [EU]

Seizures: Clinical or subclinical disturbances of cortical function due to a sudden, abnormal, excessive, and disorganized discharge of brain cells. Clinical manifestations include abnormal motor, sensory and psychic phenomena. Recurrent seizures are usually referred to as epilepsy or "seizure disorder." [NIH]

Selenium: An element with the atomic symbol Se, atomic number 34, and atomic weight 78.96. It is an essential micronutrient for mammals and other animals but is toxic in large amounts. Selenium protects intracellular structures against oxidative damage. It is an essential component of glutathione peroxidase. [NIH]

Serum: The clear portion of any body fluid; the clear fluid moistening serous membranes. 2. blood serum; the clear liquid that separates from blood on clotting. 3. immune serum; blood serum from an immunized animal used for passive immunization; an antiserum; antitoxin, or antivenin. [EU]

Sialography: Radiography of the salivary glands or ducts following injection of contrast medium. [NIH]

Sialorrhea: Increased salivary flow. [NIH]

Sinusitis: Inflammation of a sinus. The condition may be purulent or nonpurulent, acute or chronic. Depending on the site of involvement it is known as ethmoid, frontal, maxillary, or sphenoid sinusitis. [EU]

Skeletal: Pertaining to the skeleton. [EU]

Spectrum: A charted band of wavelengths of electromagnetic vibrations obtained by refraction and diffraction. By extension, a measurable range of activity, such as the range of bacteria affected by an antibiotic (antibacterial s.) or the complete range of manifestations of a disease. [EU]

Spirometry: Measurement of volume of air inhaled or exhaled by the lung. [NIH]

Splenomegaly: Enlargement of the spleen. [EU]

Spondylitis: Inflammation of the vertebrae. [EU]

Stomach: An organ of digestion situated in the left upper quadrant of the abdomen between the termination of the esophagus and the beginning of the duodenum. [NIH]

Stomatitis: Inflammation of the oral mucosa, due to local or systemic factors which may involve the buccal and labial mucosa, palate, tongue, floor of the mouth, and the gingivae. [EU]

Substrate: A substance upon which an enzyme acts. [EU]

Surgical: Of, pertaining to, or correctable by surgery. [EU]

Sweat: The fluid excreted by the sweat glands. It consists of water containing sodium chloride, phosphate, urea, ammonia, and other waste products. [NIH]

Sympathetic: 1. pertaining to, caused by, or exhibiting sympathy. 2. a sympathetic nerve or the sympathetic nervous system. [EU]

Symptomatic: 1. pertaining to or of the nature of a symptom. 2. indicative (of a particular disease or disorder). 3. exhibiting the symptoms of a particular disease but having a different cause. 4. directed at the allying of symptoms, as symptomatic treatment. [EU]

Synovitis: Inflammation of a synovial membrane. It is usually painful, particularly on motion, and is characterized by a fluctuating swelling due to effusion within a synovial sac. Synovitis is qualified as fibrinous, gonorrhoeal, hyperplastic, lipomatous, metritic, puerperal, rheumatic, scarlatinal, syphilitic, tuberculous, urethral, etc. [EU]

Systemic: Relating to a process that affects the body generally; in this instance, the way in which blood is supplied through the aorta to all body organs except the lungs. [NIH]

Teratogenic: Tending to produce anomalies of formation, or teratism (= anomaly of formation or development : condition of a monster). [EU]

Thalassemia: A group of hereditary hemolytic anemias in which there is decreased synthesis of one or more hemoglobin polypeptide chains. There are several genetic types with clinical pictures ranging from barely detectable hematologic abnormality to severe and fatal anemia. [NIH]

Thalidomide: A pharmaceutical agent originally introduced as a non-barbiturate hypnotic, but withdrawn from the market because of its known tetratogenic effects. It has been reintroduced and used for a number of immunological and inflammatory disorders. Thalidomide displays immunosuppresive and anti-angiogenic activity. It inhibits release of tumor necrosis factor alpha from monocytes, and modulates other cytokine action. [NIH]

Thoracic: Pertaining to or affecting the chest. [EU]

Thrombocytopenia: Decrease in the number of blood platelets. [EU]

Thrombophlebitis: Inflammation of a vein associated with thrombus formation. [EU]

Thyroxine: An amino acid of the thyroid gland which exerts a stimulating effect on thyroid metabolism. [NIH]

Tomography: The recording of internal body images at a predetermined plane by means of the tomograph; called also body section roentgenography. [EU]

Topical: Pertaining to a particular surface area, as a topical anti-infective applied to a certain area of the skin and affecting only the area to which it is applied. [EU]

Toxic: Pertaining to, due to, or of the nature of a poison or toxin; manifesting the symptoms of severe infection. [EU]

Toxin: A poison; frequently used to refer specifically to a protein produced by some higher plants, certain animals, and pathogenic bacteria, which is highly toxic for other living organisms. Such substances are differentiated from the simple chemical poisons and the vegetable alkaloids by their high molecular weight and antigenicity. [EU]

Toxoplasmosis: An acute or chronic, widespread disease of animals and humans caused by the obligate intracellular protozoon Toxoplasma gondii, transmitted by oocysts containing the pathogen in the feces of cats (the definitive host), usually by contaminated soil, direct exposure to infected feces, tissue cysts in infected meat, or tachyzoites (proliferating forms) in blood. [EU]

Trachea: The cartilaginous and membranous tube descending from the larynx and branching into the right and left main bronchi. [NIH]

Transplantation: The grafting of tissues taken from the patient's own body or from another. [EU]

Tuberculosis: Any of the infectious diseases of man and other animals caused by species of mycobacterium. [NIH]

Ulcer: A local defect, or excavation, of the surface of an organ or tissue; which is produced by the sloughing of inflammatory necrotic tissue. [EU]

Ulceration: 1. the formation or development of an ulcer. 2. an ulcer. [EU]

Uveitis: An inflammation of part or all of the uvea, the middle (vascular) tunic of the eye, and commonly involving the other tunics (the sclera and cornea, and the retina). [EU]

Vaccine: A suspension of attenuated or killed microorganisms (bacteria, viruses, or rickettsiae), administered for the prevention, amelioration or treatment of infectious diseases. [EU]

Vancomycin: Antibacterial obtained from Streptomyces orientalis. It is a glycopeptide related to ristocetin that inhibits bacterial cell wall assembly and is toxic to kidneys and the inner ear. [NIH]

Varicella: Chicken pox. [EU]

Vascular: Pertaining to blood vessels or indicative of a copious blood supply. [EU]

Vasculitis: Inflammation of a vessel, angiitis. [EU]

Vein: Vessel-carrying blood from various parts of the body to the heart. [NIH]

Venereal: Pertaining or related to or transmitted by sexual contact. [EU]

Ventricular: Pertaining to a ventricle. [EU]

Vestibular: Pertaining to or toward a vestibule. In dental anatomy, used to refer to the tooth surface directed toward the vestibule of the mouth. [EU]

Viral: Pertaining to, caused by, or of the nature of virus. [EU]

Viruses: Minute infectious agents whose genomes are composed of DNA or RNA, but not both. They are characterized by a lack of independent metabolism and the inability to replicate outside living host cells. [NIH]

Wheezing: Breathing with a rasp or whistling sound; a sign of airway constriction or obstruction. [NIH]

Xerostomia: Dryness of the mouth from salivary gland dysfunction, as in Sjögren's syndrome. [EU]

General Dictionaries and Glossaries

While the above glossary is essentially complete, the dictionaries listed here cover virtually all aspects of medicine, from basic words and phrases to more advanced terms (sorted alphabetically by title; hyperlinks provide rankings, information and reviews at Amazon.com):

- **Dictionary of Medical Acronymns & Abbreviations** by Stanley Jablonski (Editor), Paperback, 4th edition (2001), Lippincott Williams & Wilkins Publishers, ISBN: 1560534605,
  http://www.amazon.com/exec/obidos/ASIN/1560534605/icongroupinterna

- **Dictionary of Medical Terms : For the Nonmedical Person (Dictionary of Medical Terms for the Nonmedical Person, Ed 4)** by Mikel A. Rothenberg, M.D, et al, Paperback - 544 pages, 4th edition (2000), Barrons Educational Series, ISBN: 0764112015,
  http://www.amazon.com/exec/obidos/ASIN/0764112015/icongroupinterna

- **A Dictionary of the History of Medicine** by A. Sebastian, CD-Rom edition (2001), CRC Press-Parthenon Publishers, ISBN: 185070368X,
  http://www.amazon.com/exec/obidos/ASIN/185070368X/icongroupinterna

- **Dorland's Illustrated Medical Dictionary (Standard Version)** by Dorland, et al, Hardcover - 2088 pages, 29th edition (2000), W B Saunders Co, ISBN: 0721662544,
  http://www.amazon.com/exec/obidos/ASIN/0721662544/icongroupinterna

- **Dorland's Electronic Medical Dictionary** by Dorland, et al, Software, 29th Book & CD-Rom edition (2000), Harcourt Health Sciences, ISBN: 0721694934,
  http://www.amazon.com/exec/obidos/ASIN/0721694934/icongroupinterna

- **Dorland's Pocket Medical Dictionary (Dorland's Pocket Medical Dictionary, 26th Ed)** Hardcover - 912 pages, 26th edition (2001), W B Saunders Co, ISBN: 0721682812,
  http://www.amazon.com/exec/obidos/ASIN/0721682812/icongroupinterna /103-4193558-7304618

- **Melloni's Illustrated Medical Dictionary (Melloni's Illustrated Medical Dictionary, 4th Ed)** by Melloni, Hardcover, 4th edition (2001), CRC Press-Parthenon Publishers, ISBN: 85070094X, http://www.amazon.com/exec/obidos/ASIN/85070094X/icongroupinterna

- **Stedman's Electronic Medical Dictionary Version 5.0 (CD-ROM for Windows and Macintosh, Individual)** by Stedmans, CD-ROM edition (2000), Lippincott Williams & Wilkins Publishers, ISBN: 0781726328, http://www.amazon.com/exec/obidos/ASIN/0781726328/icongroupinterna

- **Stedman's Medical Dictionary** by Thomas Lathrop Stedman, Hardcover - 2098 pages, 27th edition (2000), Lippincott, Williams & Wilkins, ISBN: 068340007X, http://www.amazon.com/exec/obidos/ASIN/068340007X/icongroupinterna

- **Tabers Cyclopedic Medical Dictionary (Thumb Index)** by Donald Venes (Editor), et al, Hardcover - 2439 pages, 19th edition (2001), F A Davis Co, ISBN: 0803606540, http://www.amazon.com/exec/obidos/ASIN/0803606540/icongroupinterna

INDEX

A

Abdomen ... 37, 94, 99, 139, 263, 273, 279
Abscess............................110, 115, 267
Acetaminophen..............................135
Algorithms 104
Alveolitis 13, 16, 20, 21, 87
Analgesic................................. 139, 261
Anemia 118, 120, 150, 275, 280
Anergy.. 21, 76
Anesthesia....................................110
Angioedema 108
Antibiotic.................56, 85, 115, 267, 279
Antibodies..............................21, 96, 180
Antibody 32, 34, 35, 96, 97, 262, 266, 272
Antigen ... 21, 35, 55, 85, 96, 99, 261, 262, 272
Antimicrobial 124
Antineoplastic ... 34, 35, 99, 266, 268, 273
Anxiety...175
Apnea 110
Aqueous 133
Arrhythmia 45
Arteries...............................89, 130, 262
Arthropathy 102
Aspiration 110
Assay................................87, 98, 176
Asymptomatic.......................84, 96, 136
Atrophy 111, 150
Autoimmunity..................................41

B

Benign. 110, 116, 118, 120, 270, 274, 278
Benzodiazepines 110
Berylliosis......................................15
Beryllium 15, 33, 193, 263
Bilateral 75, 119, 193, 277
Biliary 44
Biochemical 91, 105, 133, 276
Biopsy 76, 80, 109, 136, 257, 258, 259
Blindness............................16, 33, 264
Bronchiectasis 110
Bronchoscope......................18, 221, 264
Buccal 78, 90, 91, 120, 264, 272, 279

C

Calcitonin 193
Capsules 191
Carbohydrates 187, 188, 198, 264
Carcinoma 108, 110, 179
Cardiac.............................118, 193, 275
Cataract...................................33, 264
Caustic..95

(C continued)

Chancre 108
Chemotherapy 29, 95, 179, 180
Chloroquine 20
Cholangitis 112
Cholecystitis 112
Cholesterol .. 116, 188, 190, 198, 265, 269
Chromosomal 81
Cirrhosis.................................. 44, 112
Cisplatin 99, 265
Collagen.......99, 104, 115, 133, 139, 265, 268, 271
Constipation 131
Cornea................................16, 37, 281
Corticosteroids ..19, 20, 28, 63, 74, 76, 85, 136
Cryoglobulinemia 104
Cryptococcosis 60
Cutaneous . 74, 76, 91, 111, 119, 272, 275
Cyclophosphamide....................... 20, 63
Cytokines 21, 86, 87
Cytomegalovirus 22, 195
Cytotoxic.............................74, 75, 180

D

Degenerative 118, 119, 189, 274, 278
Dehydration 124
Dermatology 176
Diarrhea 131, 188
Digestion............................36, 124, 279
Discoid 85, 108
Diverticulitis 112
Dysplasia 150
Dyspnea...............................11, 16, 96
Dystrophy 102, 150

E

Efficacy 90, 267
Electrolyte 119, 276
Endogenous 21
Enzyme.... 18, 76, 97, 100, 105, 108, 111, 168, 177, 178, 181, 221, 261, 273, 279
Epidemiological...............................43
Erythema... 11, 16, 85, 108, 111, 193, 195
Erythrocytes 90, 114, 180, 261, 267
Exogenous 21, 34, 81, 267

F

Fatal 14, 120, 134, 280
Fatigue.......................12, 74, 131, 262
Fetus...189
Fibroblasts.....................................94
Fibrosis 13, 14, 16, 17, 19, 21, 26, 36, 55, 63, 77, 85, 87, 96, 97, 110, 112, 124, 180, 265, 278

Fluorouracil..95
G
Gait..135
Gallium 18, 30, 258
Gastritis...112
Gastrointestinal...........111, 116, 133, 268
Glomerular.......................................130
Glomerulonephritis 77, 103
Gout..102
Granulomas 11, 14, 15, 16, 17, 18, 20,
    28, 45, 46, 47, 48, 62, 76, 77, 84, 88,
    96, 97, 111, 136, 178
H
Heartbeat 45, 55, 262
Hemoptysis..96
Hepatic..74
Hepatitis 44, 103, 104, 112
Heredity...14
Herpes 108, 116, 269
Histamine 98
Histocompatibility 103
Homeostasis......................................77
Hormonal...110
Humoral.......................................21, 97
Hypercalcemia 76, 77, 111, 130, 195
Hyperlipoproteinemia.........................102
Hypertension 103, 116, 131, 175, 270
Hyperthermia 95
Hyperthyroidism 116, 270
Hypothyroidism 117, 270
I
Iatrogenic 110
Idiopathic . 36, 63, 116, 136, 180, 270, 278
Immunotherapy 95
Impetigo 108
Induration 78, 92, 278
Infiltration.................................75, 130
Insulin 103, 117, 271
Intermittent 63
Interstitial..................26, 55, 92, 265, 278
Intestinal...............................178, 188
Intravenous 63
Invasive 136
Iodine 168, 273
Iridocyclitis.......................................75
Isotretinoin 193
K
Keloid..136
L
Lavage .. 18, 21, 79, 81, 87, 108, 111, 176
Legionellosis....................................110
Leprosy 195
Lesion 34, 35, 110, 111, 255, 259, 267,
    275
Leucine 97, 98
Lipodystrophy 112

Lubrication........................124, 126, 272
Lumbar...60
Lupus 33, 85, 102, 108, 111, 124, 136,
    265
Lymph.. 11, 15, 17, 35, 36, 62, 75, 77, 84,
    91, 97, 98, 111, 120, 130, 131, 178,
    193, 253, 272, 278
Lymphocytic 87
Lymphoma 15, 132, 177, 178, 179, 195
Lymphopenia 111
M
Maculopapular.................................111
Malaise 74
Membrane....... 33, 56, 91, 117, 118, 120,
    265, 273, 274, 278, 280
Meningitis...............................117, 273
Methotrexate 20, 89, 133, 181
Microbiology 81
Molecular 22, 92, 140, 145, 148, 149,
    277, 281
Monocytes............ 92, 178, 199, 273, 280
Mononucleosis................... 195, 199, 273
Mucosa...........78, 91, 120, 272, 273, 279
N
Nasal 91, 272
Nausea 131
Necrosis...................36, 62, 92, 278, 280
Neoplasms .102, 109, 111, 114, 118, 262,
    274
Neoplastic 94
Nephrology 103
Nephrons 77
Nephropathy 77, 103
Niacin..188
Nitrogen 34, 95, 131, 266
O
Ocular 74, 75, 133
Optic 17
Osteoarthritis 102
Osteonecrosis..................................102
Osteoporosis 102
Otorhinolaryngology 110
Otosclerosis..............................118, 275
Overdose 189
P
Pacemaker 118, 275
Palliative..75
Pancreas 103, 117, 271
Papule 115, 117, 264, 272
Paralysis 17, 36, 275
Parotitis...109
Pathogenesis.................74, 85, 111, 194
Pathologic 91, 104, 139, 276, 277
Penicillamine 20
Pentoxifylline 62
Phenotype 87

Physiologic 81, 92, 277
Pilocarpine...124
Pneumonia 30
Pneumonitis..15
Postoperative....................................110
Potassium........................103, 131, 190
Prednisone 19, 63, 75
Prevalence 12, 83, 84
Proctitis...113
Progressive 45, 69, 85, 130, 131, 136, 274
Proteins 18, 32, 34, 35, 87, 100, 115, 188, 190, 262, 266, 267, 272, 274
Psoriasis............................136, 139, 277
Pulmonary ..10, 17, 26, 49, 63, 74, 75, 85, 87, 90, 97, 110, 116, 125, 133, 175, 176, 178, 179, 180, 194, 195, 269, 270
Pyogenic 108

R
Radioactivity 18
Radiography 109
Radiotherapy 29, 95
Receptor.........................33, 85, 96, 262
Reflex...102
Reflux 103, 112
Remission.........................89, 133, 181
Renovascular...................103, 116, 270
Respiratory 16, 22, 43, 44, 55, 86, 106, 110, 111, 120, 261, 278
Retina 16, 37, 119, 278, 281
Rheumatoid 15, 22, 33, 102, 124, 133, 265
Riboflavin 188

S
Sclera............................. 16, 37, 75, 281
Sclerosis...........................77, 102, 150
Sedimentation 85
Selenium 190
Serum 18, 36, 63, 76, 79, 97, 111, 176, 177, 178, 181, 195, 257, 279
Sialography.............................. 109, 111
Sialorrhea..109
Sinusitis...........................110, 120, 279
Skeletal 74
Spectrum............................45, 79, 134
Spirometry 85

Splenomegaly...........................118, 275
Stomach.............. 20, 114, 116, 263, 268
Stomatitis 108
Substrate.................................... 97, 98
Surgical... 35, 95, 110, 118, 119, 274, 275
Sympathetic..............................102, 279
Symptomatic.................... 74, 92, 94, 280
Synovitis.. 102
Syphilis 108, 115, 264
Systemic 21, 22, 33, 36, 55, 74, 76, 81, 102, 103, 104, 109, 110, 120, 124, 125, 130, 131, 136, 178, 261, 265, 278, 279

T
Tears 132
Teratogenic 133, 198, 271
Testis................................ 168, 180, 267
Thalidomide..85
Thermoregulation.............................. 188
Thoracic..84
Thrombocytopenia 176, 178
Thyroxine 190
Tomography 111
Topical 74, 92, 94, 136, 198, 271, 280
Toxic...28, 33, 36, 85, 103, 121, 132, 139, 189, 199, 264, 275, 279, 280, 281
Toxin... 37, 280
Transplantation 41, 44, 49, 77, 103
Tuberculosis 15, 26, 85, 91, 110, 272

U
Ulcer 20, 85, 281
Ulceration 94
Uveitis............................... 91, 111, 271

V
Vaccine 133
Vascular.. 37, 55, 103, 104, 114, 261, 281
Vasculitis............................ 74, 102, 103
Vein 18, 69, 120, 280
Venereal.. 120
Ventricular...45
Viral 22, 28, 104, 109, 110
Viruses 21, 91, 140, 273, 281

W
Wheezing 96

X
Xerostomia 109, 124

Printed in the United States
27755LVS00003B/7-8

9 780597 831560